T0296397

Oncological PET/CT with Histological Confirmation

Juliano Cerci • Stefano Fanti
Dominique Delbeke

Editors

Oncological PET/CT with Histological Confirmation

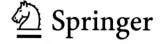

Editors
Juliano Cerci
PET/CT Center
Quanta Diagnóstico e Terapia
Curitiba
Paraná
Brazil

Dominique Delbeke
Radiology and Radiological Sciences
Vanderbilt University Medical Center
Nashville, Tennessee
USA

Stefano Fanti
Ospedale S. Orsola Malpighi
Universitary Hospital
Bologna
Italy

ISBN 978-3-319-27878-0   ISBN 978-3-319-27880-3   (eBook)
DOI 10.1007/978-3-319-27880-3

Library of Congress Control Number: 2016937004

Springer Cham Heidelberg New York Dordrecht London

© Springer International Publishing 2016
This work is subject to copyright. All rights are reserved by the Publisher, whether the whole or part of the material is concerned, specifically the rights of translation, reprinting, reuse of illustrations, recitation, broadcasting, reproduction on microfilms or in any other physical way, and transmission or information storage and retrieval, electronic adaptation, computer software, or by similar or dissimilar methodology now known or hereafter developed.
The use of general descriptive names, registered names, trademarks, service marks, etc. in this publication does not imply, even in the absence of a specific statement, that such names are exempt from the relevant protective laws and regulations and therefore free for general use.
The publisher, the authors and the editors are safe to assume that the advice and information in this book are believed to be true and accurate at the date of publication. Neither the publisher nor the authors or the editors give a warranty, express or implied, with respect to the material contained herein or for any errors or omissions that may have been made.

Printed on acid-free paper

Springer International Publishing AG Switzerland is part of Springer Science+Business Media (www.springer.com)

Preface

Many books on positron emission tomography (PET)/computed tomography (CT) have been published in recent years, reflecting the well-established role of PET/CT in the many steps of oncological patients care. PET/CT results often guide or lead to changes in therapy. The positive findings should first be confirmed by histology. Furthermore, most guidelines that include PET/CT recommend biopsy prior to changes in therapy. PET/CT-guided biopsy offers a feasible new approach of potential value in optimizing the diagnostic yield of biopsies.

This book, *Oncological PET/CT with Histological Confirmation*, takes into account that when a suspicious neoplastic lesion is found, a biopsy for histological characterization is fundamental in most scenarios. Early and accurate histologic diagnosis of a neoplastic condition usually leads to the more appropriate treatment and improves the chances of cure.

In the 1990s, ^{18}F-FDG PET oncological clinical applications emerged and are now the most common indication. ^{18}F-FDG PET is well established for the evaluation of several ^{18}F-FDG-avid malignancies.

PET/CT results often guide or lead to changes in therapy. The positive findings should whenever possible be confirmed by histology. In that sense, PET/CT-guided biopsy offers a feasible new approach of potential value in optimizing the diagnostic yield of biopsies. Also, PET/CT-guided biopsy could be especially indicated in patients with only metabolic lesion but no anatomic correspondent lesion, in whom tumor transformation/mutation is suspected, or in patients with new multiple lesions in a patient not known to have malignancy or who has had a prolonged remission or more than one primary malignancy.

Chapters 1 to 3 describe a bit of history of image-guided biopsy, the technical procedure of ^{18}F-FDG PET/CT-guided biopsy, and possible acute complications of biopsy procedures.

All other chapters describe clinical applications of ^{18}F-FDG PET/CT studies and emphasize the importance of histological documentation.

Redondo et al. describe the use of ^{18}F-FDG PET/CT for guiding biopsy in lymphoma patients, since ^{18}F-FDG PET/CT has rapidly become the preferred imaging modality for lymphoma evaluation. The clinical indications include initial staging, assessment of early metabolic response to treatment, evaluation of prognosis, end-treatment response assessment, and early detection of disease recurrence. Biopsy-guided ^{18}F-FDG PET/CT plays an important role in histological transformation of indolent lymphoma and in detection of bone marrow involvement.

Ceci et al. focus the use choline PET/CT in prostate cancer patients. The authors emphasize the molecular imaging advantages compared to conventional imaging techniques in intra-prostatic cancer.

Zanoni et al. report the use of FLT PET/CT-guided biopsy in the evaluation of cancer, as deregulated cell cycle progression is a hallmark of cancer. FLT has been developed as a surrogate PET marker of cellular proliferation and is presented as an alternative to ^{18}F-FDG, a biomarker of glucose metabolism associated with false positive findings in inflammatory processes.

Cerci et al. describe ^{18}F-FDG PET/CT-guided biopsy in pancreatic lesions. Pancreatic cancer represents an important cause of cancer mortality, probably related to its usual delayed diagnosis and aggressive characteristics. The interest in proper evaluation of pancreatic lesions and unveiling their histological aspects has been growing strong over the last years.

Finally, Nani et al. describe the role of ^{18}F-FDG PET/CT for bone and soft tissue biopsy, as in the clinical practice, it is quite common to diagnose a bone or soft tissue lesion that is amenable to biopsy. This is particularly true in patients who come to the hospital with a history of cancer, with radiological signs consistent with malignancy, or with the suspicion of focal septic inflammation.

Written by a team of renowned international experts, the three editors are expert nuclear medicine physicians from Europe and North and South America, and the range of experiences gained in using PET/CT across the globe is reflected in this book.

Curitiba, Brazil   Juliano Cerci
Bologna, Italy   Stefano Fanti
Nashville, TN, USA   Dominique Delbeke

Contents

History of Image-Guided Biopsy

Juliano J. Cerci, Mateos Bogoni,
and Dominique Delbeke

When a suspicious lesion is found during a physical or imaging exam, histological characterization is frequently required. Early and accurate histologic diagnosis of a neoplastic condition requires tissue sampling and leads to the appropriate treatment.

The term biopsy derives from the Greek language, *bio* referring to "life" and *opsias* meaning "to see." It was first used by a French dermatologist, Ernest Besnier, in 1879 [1]. Biopsy technique consists of obtaining tissue samples for further pathological investigation. It is basically divided into *excisional biopsy*, where a whole suspicious lesion is removed, and *incisional biopsy*, where only one part is sampled. Generally, incisional biopsy is performed with different-sized needles (gauges), with or without guidance of an imaging method such as conventional radiography, ultrasonography (US), computerized tomography (CT), magnetic resonance imaging (MRI), and, more recently, integrated positron emission tomography/computerized tomography (PET/CT).

The first report of suspicious masses being accessed with the aid of needles is found in the treatise *Kitab al-Tasrif* (The Method of Medicine), written by Arab physician Abu al-Qasim Khalaf ibn al-Abbas Al-Zahrawi, famously known as Albucasis (936–1013 AD) [2]. In his works, he discusses therapeutic puncturing of different types of thyroid goiter.

Entering the field of diagnosis per se, although literature from the late nineteenth century is rather limited [3], Kun [4] was presumably the first to describe percutaneous biopsy being performed with needles in his work entitled, *A new instrument for the diagnosis of tumors* (1847). At the dawn of the twentieth century, needle biopsy became more common in main health centers around the globe. The fact that the procedures were blindly performed resulted in higher rates of severe complications (such as pneumothorax and internal bleeding) and occasional deaths. Not surprisingly, percutaneous biopsy faced great criticism from the medical community at the time.

Hopper [3] highlights the great advances in percutaneous needle biopsy after the integration of imaging methods, especially after World War I. The use of fluoroscopy to localize and remove shrapnel in battlefield hospitals might be considered the initial step toward the successful partnership between imaging techniques and invasive medical procedures [5]. Hopper [3] describes the first reports of imaging tests (fluoroscopy) being applied in the guidance of biopsies. Blady [6],

J.J. Cerci (✉) • M. Bogoni
Quanta – Diagnóstico e Terapia, Curitiba, PR, Brazil
e-mail: cercijuliano@hotmail.com; bogonimateos@gmail.com

D. Delbeke
Radiology and Radiological Sciences, Vanderbilt University Medical Center, Nashville, TN, USA
e-mail: dominique.delbeke@vanderbilt.edu

© Springer International Publishing 2016
J. Cerci et al. (eds.), *Oncological PET/CT with Histological Confirmation*,
DOI 10.1007/978-3-319-27880-3_1

physician at the Memorial Hospital in New York, reported 27 percutaneous biopsies performed with fluoroscopy guidance. This exam permitted localizing the suspicious lesion in two planes. Martin, Ellis, and Stewart became strong needle biopsy supporters at the beginning of the decade, with their percutaneous biopsy experience of 10,000 patients in a 4-year period [7–9].

Percutaneous biopsy and imaging techniques continue to develop today. From the 27 biopsied lesions reported in Blady's work, 19 were confined to the chest and 8 to the bones [6]. The reported success rate of lung biopsy jumped from 40 % in 1931, when the procedures were blindly performed, to 90 % in 1937, with the aid of imaging guidance. There was also a decrease in the number of complications [10, 11].

By the early 1950s, successful brain, vertebral column, and kidney biopsies (the last one with pioneer utilization of intravenous contrast methods) were reported [12–16]. In the 1970s, the introduction of significantly thinner needles allowed much safer biopsies, with drastic reduction in the complication rates [17].

In the same decade, image-guided biopsy had a major breakthrough: the development of cross-sectional techniques. Doctor Kenneth D. Hopper said: "With the possible exception of the use of fluoroscopy to control the biopsy procedure, no other development or technique has had a greater impact on radiographically guided percutaneous biopsy than has cross-sectional imaging" [3]. US and CT rapidly became important tools in the guidance of percutaneous biopsies, greatly improving the accuracy of diagnosis and staging of cancer and improving therapeutic decisions [18].

Patient preparation includes local anesthesia and the possibility of intravenous light or profound sedation [18]. Low platelet count or coagulation abnormalities are relative contraindications for biopsy procedure. The imaging method of choice for guiding the biopsy depends on factors such as accuracy, availability, cost, and safety. After performing the biopsy, pathologists analyze samples, and from their findings, diagnosis is established. Image-guided percutaneous biopsy sensitivity varies according to the site being sampled and the imaging method used for guidance [18].

1.1 Ultrasound-Guided Biopsy

Ultrasonography is a common method used for guiding biopsies [3]. It became popular after the introduction of a proper US aspiration transducer in 1972 [19]. US is widely applied in percutaneous needle biopsy, particularly in superficial soft tissue [20] and abdominal lesions, such as kidney, liver, and pancreas [21]. The advantage is no radiation and the widespread availability of the procedure. However, US also presents some well-known limitations, such as poor visualization of deep structures in the presence of air or bones, as well as in overweight patients (due to the soft tissue attenuation) [3].

1.2 CT-Guided Biopsy

Given these limitations, CT is commonly used to guide biopsy. Allan MacLeod Cormack (1924–1998) and Godfrey Newbold Hounsfield (1919–2004) both contributed to the development of CT [22]. Cormack, working as a theoretical physicist at Harvard University in the early 1960s, developed the concept of X-ray projection reconstruction. Hounsfield developed the first CT scan, working for EMI Ltd. at the company's central research laboratories. The two scientists won the Nobel Prize for Physiology or Medicine in 1979, for their role on the development of CT.

Hounsfield was well experienced with computer programming as he served Great Britain during World War II, developing their radar air defense systems. In the late 1960s, he started assembling the first CT prototype at EMI, whereas major imaging companies believed that the computer technology at the time was not sufficiently developed for the fast calculus required [23]. Initially, Hounsfield scanned animal organs, such as brains and kidneys of pigs. In 1968, he patented computerized tomography. At the time, image acquisition was as long as 20 min, and their reconstruction through computer calculus could take as long as days.

It took 3 years for CT to be applied in clinical practice. Partnering with neurologist James Ambrose, at Atkinson Morley Hospital in

Wimbledon, Hounsfield and his team performed the very first patient CT scan on October 1, 1971. The prototype used was the EMI Mark I, developed for head scanning only. The patient was a woman with a suspected brain tumor [22]. After seeing the resulting image, Hounsfield said "My God, it does work – I can see the tumor just as I always hoped" [23]. With this CT prototype, scan time was of approximately 4.5 min, reconstruction of the image 20 s, and the slice thickness was around 13 mm [22].

The interest in expanding this novel technology to other medical specialties was immediate, as well as the interest of other companies in competing with EMI in the CT business. By 1975, EMI, Siemens, and GE were already selling different CT scanner models, and the investigations for improvements were at full throttle. Several other small companies were acquired by the large ones, and competition was relentless. By 1975, full-body scans were already available when GE presented a new generation of CT scanners: the fan-beam scanners associated with multiple detectors. This innovation decreased scanning time to around 5 s, and the quality of imaging improved greatly [23].

By allowing proper visualization of deeper structures, radiologists were able to sample tissues at sites considered inaccessible at the time. The feasibility of CT-guided biopsy was rapidly unraveled. Alfidi (1975) [24] was the first to report the procedure and performed to biopsy a retroperitoneal mass.

In the late 1980s, the single-slice helical CT scanner was introduced [25]. The scanner was able to perform a helical movement by making modifications to the electrical conduction machinery. This implied faster scanning, and the images were reconstructed from a continuous "helix" of data instead of multiple "pies." The helical technique offered better images, but it was not great for moving objects or for covering large longitudinal areas [25].

This problem was solved in the late 1990s, with the introduction of multi-slice helical CT scanners, with multiple rows of detectors. Using this technology, several overlapped helixes supply the computer for imaging reconstruction [25].

State-of-the-art scanners have up to 320 separated channels (helixes), providing significantly thinner slices in comparison with old single-slice scanners.

With the development of multi-slice CT technology, CT-guided biopsy (as well as other types of interventional radiology procedures) gained even more ground, being performed in virtually every part of the body [3]. CT stands as the main choice for accessing lung, bone, spine, and base-of-skull lesions [18].

Although the benefits outweigh the risks, CT-guided biopsy also holds its share of complications. Potential complications vary according to the site accessed. For thoracic punctures, the most common complication is pneumothorax [26], with an incidence of up to 50 % [18]. Usually, this complication is successfully managed with a conservative strategy. Large pneumothorax that requires intervention is reported in 3–15 % of cases [27]. Other risks are quite rare, such as hemothorax, hemoptysis, cardiac arrest, respiratory arrest, air embolism, and shock [26]. All complications associated to transthoracic biopsy are more likely to occur in chronic smokers [18]. For bone biopsies, complications rarely occur, usually mild hemorrhage. Vertebral column punctures can lead to neurologic complications in up to 8 % of patients [18]. For abdominal biopsies, the risk depends on the organ being accessed. In general, precautions must be taken to avoid damage to the biliary tract (especially when the liver is biopsied), as well as vascular damages, which can be life threatening. Biopsy of the pancreas has a complication rate of up to 5 % [28], the most common being hematoma and acute pancreatitis [29]. Unusual complications at other abdominal sites have also been reported, such as adrenergic crisis due to puncturing pheochromocytoma [30].

1.3 MRI-Guided Biopsy

The introduction of magnetic resonance imaging opened new doors for percutaneous needle biopsy. The first report of MRI-guided biopsy of head and neck lesions was published in 1986 by

Mueller et al. [31]. MRI-guided biopsy is considered a safe and effective procedure, presenting some unique features [32]. It is best indicated in abdominal, soft tissue, and bone biopsies, especially for lesions poorly visualized by CT or US [33]. MRI can be performed instead of CT when radiation exposure is a concern or the patient is allergic to iodinated contrast agents. Specific indications for MRI-guided biopsy are for subdiaphragmatic lesions (which can be difficult to access through CT due to angulation problems) and for bone marrow edema of unknown origin (where MRI offers the best visualization) [32]. It is important to highlight that MRI-guided percutaneous biopsy requires special instruments, due to the magnetic field created by the scanning process.

As for any imaging method, there are limitations for the MRI-guided biopsy procedure. Proper access to suspicious lesions might be restricted by its size and by image artifacts created by the equipment. In addition, for chest lesions, MRI guidance is generally contraindicated due to poor visualization of pneumothorax formation, which is the main complication of thoracic puncturing [32].

1.4 PET/CT-Guided Biopsy

PET/CT-guided biopsy is another alternative for FDG-avid lesions combining the well-established value of anatomical information from CT with PET metabolic characterization [34]. To understand how PET and CT are being currently applied together in biopsy procedures, first we must understand how PET technology was created.

The existence of positrons, or "positive electrons," was demonstrated in the 1930s [35]. When a positron and an electron interact, they emit two photons 180° apart in the process of annihilation. Sweet et al. [35] reported the use of positron detectors for localization of brain tumors with positron-emitting radionuclides through the coincidence principle in 1951. Coincidence detection by PET scanners allows creation of PET emission images. Most PET radiotracers are produced by cyclotrons developed in the 1930s and 1940s, which principles are still used in the radiopharmaceutical industry today.

The first PET human tomography was built in 1974 through the work of Phelps et al. [36]. This prototype had 48 detectors, while the most modern PET scanners have hundreds of thousands of detectors (up to approximately 120,000) [36]. The first images obtained with PET techniques were published in 1975, using a filtered back projection algorithm developed by Ter-Pogossian, Phelps, and Hoffman [37]. The PET radiopharmaceuticals were ^{15}O-oxygen, ^{11}C-glucose, and ^{18}F-fluorideand, and the first published images showed blood flow, oxygen, and glucose metabolism in the brain, in addition to fluoride consumption by the bones [38, 39].

^{18}F-fluorodeoxyglucose (^{18}F-FDG) is the most commonly used PET radiopharmaceutical and was first synthetized in 1978 by Ido et al. [40]. ^{18}F has the ability of being incorporated in molecules of interest (in this case, glucose) in place of hydrogen atoms or hydroxyl groups without significantly altering their biological function. Furthermore, its half-life time is relatively long (110 min) [41]. In 1977, Sokoloff et al. [42] described the procedure for measurement of local cerebral glucose utilization with ^{14}C-deoxyglucose. Two years later, Reivich and colleagues published the procedure to measure regional glucose metabolism with ^{18}F-FDG [43]. Phelps et al. [44] acquired the first PET images using ^{18}F-FDG. In the 1980s, the first ^{18}F-FDG PET clinical applications were related to brain functional mapping and myocardial viability. Several "PET centers" were created, specially focusing in the development of a cardiac clinical PET imaging for the diagnosis of coronary artery disease.

In the 1990s, ^{18}F-FDG PET clinical applications emerged and are now the most common indication. Otto Warburg et al. (1924) discovered that cancer cells exhibit increased rate of glycolysis [45]. Glycolysis is a basic biochemical pathway for ATP production, which is usually present in normal cells under hypoxemic conditions. In most of cancer cells, however, glycolysis is present even in an oxygen-rich environment, and neoplasms show elevated glucose consumption. In the early 1980s, Di Chiro et al. [46] demonstrated that brain tumors accumulate ^{18}F-FDG and their degree of malignancy was proportional to the uptake degree. In 1991, Phelps et al. [47] published the first whole-body oncology images and the April issue of *The Journal of Nuclear Medicine* cover stated: "Clinical PET: Its Time Has Come." Reimbursement for ^{18}F-FDG PET procedures became available in the USA at the end of the twentieth century.

^{18}F-FDG PET is now well established for evaluation of ^{18}F-FDG-avid malignancies [41, 48, 49]. Gambhir et al. [50] found an overall ^{18}F-FDG PET's average sensitivity of 84 % and specificity of 88 % for cancer detection.

Large malignant lesions can be heterogeneous and ^{18}F-FDG PET/CT is able to guide biopsy to the area of highest ^{18}F-FDG uptake [34, 51].

The first studies on ^{18}F-FDG PET/CT-guided biopsy were published in 2008 by O'Sullivan et al. in musculoskeletal lesions [52]. Klaeser et al. [51] published their initial experiences with 12 patients with various malignancies (breast cancer, non-small-cell lung cancer, cervical cancer, soft tissue sarcoma, and osteosarcoma). The team obtained representative samples in 92 % of the cases, without major complications. Govindarajan et al. [54] published their results and came to the same conclusions. Tatli et al. [53] obtained good diagnostic results for PET/CT-guided biopsies of abdominal lesions (liver, presacral soft tissue, retroperitoneal lymph nodes, spleen, and pancreas). Klaeser et al. [55] reported a 56 % clinical impact rate (changing in therapeutic management) due to PET/CT-guided biopsy in 20 patients with active bone lesions. Werner et al. [56] published a case report where FDG-PET/CT-guided biopsy revealed bone metastases of a neuroendocrine small-cell cancer of unknown origin after MRI and CT results were inconclusive, which altered the patient's clinical management. Venkatesan et al. [57] reported 33 percutaneous and 3 intraoperative biopsies of 36 ^{18}F-FDG-avid lesions with real-time FDG-PET guidance. Thirty-one of these 36 biopsies were diagnostic. The study also evaluated radiofrequency ablation using multimodality image fusion.

In 2012, our group reported 130 lesions accessed through PET/CT guidance in several body sites, obtaining representative tissue samples in 98.5 % of the total. Of the 130 lesions, 18 % (23/180) were referred to PET/CT after a non-diagnostic CT-guided biopsy. Malignancy was diagnosed after PET/CT-guided biopsy in 21/23 lesions [52]. Similar results were obtained by Purandare et al. [54] in a study with 122 patients in 2013.

The publication of several additional studies [34, 51, 58, 59] consolidates the great value of PET/CT as the imaging method of choice for guiding biopsy procedures. Novel PET radiopharmaceuticals are also being investigated for guiding biopsies [51, 60].

Dr. Henry N. Wagner, Jr. [35], stated in 1998: "In the present climate of changing medical practice, it is increasingly clear that ignorance is what is expensive in medicine. Better selection of patients for specific therapy, whether it is surgery, radiation, or chemotherapy, and better monitoring the effect of therapy is where revolutionary advances are being made. History repeats itself, because no one listens the first time. The messages being sent by the pioneers in the development of PET are now being heard loud and clear."

References

1. Zerbino DD. Biopsy: its history, current and future outlook. Lik Sprava. 1994;(3–4):1–9. Review. Russian. PubMed.
2. Diamantis A, Magiorkinis E, Koutselini H. Fine-needle aspiration (FNA) biopsy: historical aspects. Folia Histochem Cytobiol. 2009;47(2):191–7.
3. Hopper KD. Percutaneous, radiographically guided biopsy: a history. Radiology. 1995;196:329–33.
4. Kun M. A new instrument for the diagnosis of tumors. Mon J Med Sci. 1847;7:853–4.
5. Skinner EH. The Sutton method of foreign body localization. Am J Roentgenology. 1917;4:350–5.
6. Blady JV. Aspiration biopsy of tumors in obscure or difficult locations under roentgenoscopic guidance. AJR. 1939;42:515–24.
7. Stewart FW. The diagnosis of tumors by aspiration. Am J Pathol. 1933;9:801–12.
8. Martin HE, Effis EB. Aspiration biopsy. Surg Gynecol Obstet. 1934;59:578–89.
9. Martin HE, Stewart FW. The advantages and limitations of aspiration biopsy. AJR. 1936;35:245–7.

10. Craver LF, Binkley JS. Aspiration biopsy of tumors of the lung. J Thorac Surg. 1939;8:436–63.
11. Craver LF. Diagnosis of malignant lung tumors by aspiration biopsy and by sputum examination. Surgery. 1940;8:947–60.
12. Iversen F, Bran C. Aspiration biopsy of the kidney. Am J Med. 1951;11:324–30.
13. Lusted LB, Mortimore GE, Hopper J. Needle renal biopsy under image amplifier control. AJR. 1956; 75:953–5.
14. Lindblom K. Diagnostic kidney puncture in cysts and tumors. AJR. 1952;68:209–15.
15. Peirce CB, Cone WV, Bouchard J, Lewis RC. Medulloblastoma: non-operative management with roentgen therapy after aspiration biopsy. Radiology. 1949;52:621–32.
16. Mazet R, Cozen L. The diagnostic value of vertebral needle biopsy. Ann Surg. 1952;135:245–52.
17. Zornoza J, Snow J, Lukeman JM, Libshitz HI. Aspiration biopsy of discrete pulmonary lesions using a new thin needle. Radiology. 1977;123:519–20.
18. Interventional Radiology Grand Rounds. Society of Interventional Radiology. 2004 – www.SIRweb.org.
19. Goldberg BB, Pollack HM. Ultrasonic aspiration transducer. Radiology. 1972;102:187–9.
20. Soudack M, Nachtigal A, Vladovski E, Brook O, Gaitini D. Sonographically guided percutaneous needle biopsy of soft tissue masses with histopathologic correlation. J Ultrasound Med. 2006;25(10):1271–7.
21. Wang J, Gao L, Tang S, Li T, Lei Y, Xie H, Liang J, Chen B, Wang X, Fan D. A retrospective analysis on the diagnostic value of ultrasound-guided percutaneous biopsy for peritoneal lesions. World J Surg Oncol. 2013;11(1):251.
22. Cierniak R. Some words about the history of computed tomography. In: X-ray computed tomography in biomedical engineering. London: Springer-Verlag London Limited; 2011. p. 7–19. doi: 10.1007/978-0-85729-027-4.
23. Robb WL. Perspective on the first 10 years of the CT scanner industry. Acad Radiol. 2003;10(7):756–60. PubMed.
24. Alfidi RJ, Haaga J, Meaney TF, et al. Computed tomography of the thorax and abdomen; a preliminary report. Radiology. 1975;117:257–64.
25. Wesolowski JR, Lev MH. CT: history, technology, and clinical aspects. Semin Ultrasound CT MR. 2005;26(6):376–9. PubMed.
26. Tomiyama N, Yasuhara Y, Nakajima Y, Adachi S, Arai Y, Kusumoto M, Eguchi K, Kuriyama K, Sakai F, Noguchi M, Murata K, Murayama S, Mochizuki T, Mori K, Yamada K. CT-guided needle biopsy of lung lesions: a survey of severe complication based on 9783 biopsies in Japan. Eur J Radiol. 2006;59(1): 60–4.
27. Lal H, Neyaz Z, Nath A, Borah S. CT-guided percutaneous biopsy of intrathoracic lesions. Korean J Radiol. 2012;13(2):210–26. Published online 2012 March 7.
28. Paulsen SD, Nghiem HV, Negussie E, Higgins EJ, Caoili EM, Francis IR. Evaluation of imaging-guided core biopsy of pancreatic masses. AJR Am J Roentgenol. 2006;187(3):769–72.
29. Mueller P, Miketic L, Simeone J, et al. Severe acute pancreatitis after percutaneous biopsy of the pancreas. AJR. 1988;151:493–4.
30. Koenker R, Mueller P, vanSonnenberg E. Interventional radiology of the adrenal glands. Semin Roentgenol. 1988;22:314–22.
31. Mueller PR, Stark DD, Simeone JF, et al. MR-guided aspiration biopsy: needle design and clinical trials. Radiology. 1986;161:605–9.
32. Adam G, Bücker A, Nolte-Ernsting C, Tacke J, Günther RW. Interventional MR imaging: percutaneous abdominal and skeletal biopsies and drainages of the abdomen. Eur Radiol. 1999;9(8):1471–8.
33. Kerimaa P, Marttila A, Hyvönen P, Ojala R, Lappi-Blanco E, Tervonen O, Blanco Sequeiros R. MRI-guided biopsy and fine needle aspiration biopsy (FNAB) in the diagnosis of musculoskeletal lesions. Eur J Radiol. 2013;82(12):2328–33.
34. Kobayashi K, Bhargava P, Raja S, Nasseri F, Al-Balas HA, Smith DD, George SP, Vij MS. Image-guided biopsy: what the interventional radiologist needs to know about PET/CT. Radiographics. 2012;32(5): 1483–501.
35. Wagner Jr HN. A brief history of positron emission tomography (PET). Semin Nucl Med. 1998;28(3):213–20. PubMed PMID: 9704363.
36. Nutt R. The history of positron emission tomography. Mol Imag Biol. 2002;4:11–26.
37. Ter-Pogossian MM, Phelps ME, Hoffman EJ, et al. A positron-emission transaxial tomograph for nuclear imaging (PETT). Radiology. 1975;114:89–98.
38. Hoffmann EJ, Phelps ME, Mullani NA, Higgins CS, Ter-Pogossian MM. Design and performance characteristics of a whole-body transaxial tomograph. J Nucl Med. 1976;17:493–503.
39. Phelps ME, Hoffman EJ, Mullani NA, et al. Design considerations for a positron emission transaxial tomograph (PET III). IEEE Trans Biomed Eng. 1976;NS-23:516–22.
40. Ido T, Wan CN, Casella V, et al. Labeled 2-dexoy-D-glucose analogs: 18F labeled 2-deoxy-2-fluoro-D-glucose, 2-deoxy-2-fluoro-D-mannose and 14C-2-deoxy-2-fluoro-D-glucose. J Labelled Comp Radiopharm. 1978;14:175–83.
41. Kelloff GJ, Hoffman JM, Johnson B, Scher HI, Siegel BA, Cheng EY, Cheson BD, O'shaughnessy J, Guyton KZ, Mankoff DA, Shankar L, Larson SM, Sigman CC, Schilsky RL, Sullivan DC. Progress and promise of FDG-PET imaging for cancer patient management and oncologic drug development. Clin Cancer Res. 2005;11(8):2785–808. Review PubMed.
42. Sokoloff L, Reivich M, Kennedy C, des Rosieers MH, et al. The [14C] deoxyglucose method for the measurement of local cerebral glucose utilization: theory, proce-

dure and normal values in the conscious and anesthetized albino rat. J Neurochem. 1977;28:897–916.

43. Reivich M, Kuhl DE, Wolf A, et al. The [18F] fluoro-deoxyglucose method for the measurement of local cerebral glucose utilization in man. Circ Res. 1979; 44:127–37.

44. Phelps ME, Huang SC, Hoffman EJ, Selin C, Sokoloff L, Kuhl DE. Tomographic measurement of local cerebral glucose metabolic rate in humans with (F-18)2-fluoro-2-deoxy-D-glucose: validation of method. Ann Neurol. 1979;6(5):371–88. PubMed.

45. Warburg O, Posener K, Negelein E. Uber den stoffwechsel der carcinomzelle. Biochem Zeitschrift. 1924;152:309–35.

46. Di Chiro G, Oldfield E, Bairamian D, et al. In vivo glucose utilization of tumors of the brain stem and spinal cord. New York: Raven; 1985. p. 351–61.

47. Dahlbom M, Hoffman EJ, Hoh CK, Schiepers C, Rosenqvist G, Hawkins RA, Phelps ME. Evaluation of a positron emission tomography (PET) scanner for whole body imaging. J Nucl Med. 1992;33:1191–9.

48. Fletcher JW, Djulbegovic B, Soares HP, Siegel BA, Lowe VJ, Lyman GH, Coleman RE, Wahl R, Paschold JC, Avril N, Einhorn LH, Suh WW, Samson D, Delbeke D, Gorman M, Shields AF. Recommendations on the use of 18F-FDG PET in oncology. J Nucl Med. 2008;49(3):480–508.

49. Hain SF, Curran KM, Beggs AD, Fogelman I, O'Doherty MJ, Maisey MN. FDG-PET as a "metabolic biopsy" tool in thoracic lesions with indeterminate biopsy. Eur J Nucl Med. 2001;28(9):1336–40. PubMed.

50. Gambhir SS, Czernin J, Schwimmer J, et al. A tabulated summary of the FDGPET literature. J Nucl Med. 2001;42:1–93S.

51. Klaeser B, Mueller MD, Schmid RA, Guevara C, Krause T, Wiskirchen J. PET-CT-guided interventions in the management of FDG-positive lesions in patients suffering from solid malignancies: initial experiences. Eur Radiol. 2009;19(7):1780–5.

52. O'Sullivan PJ, Rohren EM, Madewell JE. Positron emission tomography-CT imaging in guiding musculoskeletal biopsy. Radiol Clin North Am. 2008; 46(3):475–86.

53. Tatli S, Gerbaudo VH, Mamede M, Tuncali K, Shyn PB, Silverman SG. Abdominal masses sampled at PET/CT-guided percutaneous biopsy: initial experience with registration of prior PET/CT images. Radiology. 2010;256(1):305–11.

54. Govindarajan MJ, Nagaraj KR, Kallur KG, Sridhar PS. PET/CT guidance for percutaneous fine needle aspiration cytology/biopsy. In J Radiol Imag. 2009; 19:208–9. [PubMed:19881087].

55. Klaeser B, Wiskirchen J, Wartenberg J, Weitzel T, Schmid RA, Mueller MD, Krause T. PET/CT-guided biopsies of metabolically active bone lesions: applications and clinical impact. Eur J Nucl Med Mol Imaging. 2010;37(11):2027–36.

56. Werner MK, Aschoff P, Reimold M, Pfannenberg C. FDG-PET/CT-guided biopsy of bone metastases sets a new course in patient management after extensive imaging and multiple futile biopsies. Br J Radiol. 2011;84(999):e65–7.

57. Venkatesan AM, Kadoury S, Abi-Jaoudeh N, Levy EB, Maass-Moreno R, Krücker J, Dalal S, Xu S, Glossop N, Wood BJ. Real-time FDG PET guidance during biopsies and radiofrequency ablation using multimodality fusion with electromagnetic navigation. Radiology. 2011;260(3):848–56.

58. Win AZ, Aparici CM. Real-time FDG PET/CT-guided bone biopsy in a patient with two primary malignancies. Eur J Nucl Med Mol Imaging. 2013;40(11): 1787–8.

59. Fukuda H, Kubota K, Matsuzawa T. Pioneering and fundamental achievements on the development of positron emission tomography (PET) in oncology. Tohoku J Exp Med. 2013;230(3):155–69. PubMed PMID: 23883588.

60. Dhingra VK, Mahajan A, Basu S. Emerging clinical applications of PET based molecular imaging in oncology: the promising future potential for evolving personalized cancer care. Indian J Radiol Imaging. 2015;25(4):332–41. doi: 10.4103/0971-3026.169467.

^{18}F-FDG PET/CT-Guided Biopsy: Technical Procedure

2

Juliano J. Cerci, Mateos Bogoni, and Dominique Delbeke

2.1 Introduction

Previous studies demonstrated promising results [1–10] for PET/CT-guided biopsy as an efficient diagnostic tool. In this chapter, we discuss the technical procedures to perform PET/CT-guided percutaneous biopsies.

PET/CT-guided biopsy can be performed in practically any PET/CT scanner, although, scanners with wider scanner bore diameter (>70 cm) are more suitable for large patients, in addition to allowing image acquisition with partially inserted biopsy needle or ablation devices [11]. Percutaneous biopsies can be performed safely on an outpatient basis. The suite in which PET/CT-guided biopsy is performed must follow safety measures for patient and medical staff. The procedure room must be equipped with wall gases, proper electric support, anesthesia equipment, and a code cart. Any equipment used in

typical US or CT-guided biopsy can also be used in the PET/CT suite [11].

The fusion of PET and CT images is obtained through software algorithms, in a process known as *image registration*, which requires proper image alignment [12]. Registration methods were used more often prior to the development of integrated PET/CT scans, when PET and CT images were obtained by different devices [13]. There are two basic types of image registration: rigid (linear) and nonrigid (elastic). The first one is less time consuming and demands lower-complexity computer systems. It is suitable for analyzing structures that are relatively still, such as the retroperitoneum and pelvis. The second one, though more appropriate for organs subject to respiratory or cardiac motion, is also more time consuming and requires very powerful computers (being less used, consequently, in interventional procedures) [14, 15].

It is not necessary to perform the biopsy procedure in the same institution or scanner where the PET/CT images were acquired, as long as the data set is in Digital Imaging and Communications in Medicine (DICOM) format. If the patient's position during the biopsy differs from the position in which PET/CT images were obtained, manual alignment of PET/CT images might be necessary in order to match the intraprocedural CT images [16].

For administration of the ^{18}F-FDG, a properly shielded uptake room is necessary, where the patient must remain from the time of ^{18}F-FDG injection

J.J. Cerci (✉)
Quanta – Diagnóstico e Terapia, Curitiba, PR, Brazil
e-mail: cercijuliano@hotmail.com

M. Bogoni
Hospital de Clínicas – Universidade Federal do Paraná, Curitiba, PR, Brazil
e-mail: bogonimateos@gmail.com

D. Delbeke
Radiology and Radiological Sciences, Vanderbilt University Medical Center, Nashville, TN, USA
e-mail: dominique.delbeke@vanderbilt.edu

© Springer International Publishing 2016
J. Cerci et al. (eds.), *Oncological PET/CT with Histological Confirmation*,
DOI 10.1007/978-3-319-27880-3_2

until the PET images are acquired. With a 370 MBq (10 mCi) ^{18}F-FDG administered activity, the radiation exposure to the patient is approximately twice the annual natural background exposure of a person living 1 year in the USA [17]. As the ^{18}F-FDG half-life is 110 min, a 2-h interval allows a radiation decay of almost 50 % (consequently decreasing radiation exposure to medical personnel) without compromising the level of ^{18}F-FDG uptake by the tumors (malignant tumors continue to accumulate ^{18}F-FDG over time up to 4–8 h) [18].

2.2 PET/CT-Guided Biopsy: Indications

Patients with suspicious lesions should be discussed in a multidisciplinary setting with the referring physician and an imaging physician at a minimum. Percutaneous biopsy should be considered but are not limited to patients with the following findings on imaging:

- New, or enlarging, or PET-positive solitary pulmonary lesion (>1.0 cm) which is not amenable to diagnosis by bronchoscopy, or CT shows it is unlikely to be accessible by bronchoscopy
- New, or enlarging, or PET-positive lesion (>1.0 cm) which is suspicious for malignancy (lung, hepatic, breast, pancreas, spleen, adrenal, kidney, soft tissue, bone, and lymph node)
- New multiple lesions in patients with no known malignancy or with prolonged remission or more than one primary malignancy
- Persistent pulmonary focal infiltrates either single or multiple, for which no diagnosis has been made by sputum or blood culture, serology, or bronchoscopy
- Patients in which with lymphoma, breast or lung cancer with metastatic disease and tumor transformation/mutation are suspected

2.3 PET/CT-Guided Biopsy: Contraindications

There are contraindications to biopsy and the balance of benefit against risk for the procedure should be assessed at a multidisciplinary meeting. Lack of a safe path to perform biopsy is the most common contraindication.

For the biopsy procedure, prothrombin time (PT), activated partial thromboplastin time (APTT), and platelet count should be checked preoperatively. Oral anticoagulants should be stopped before biopsy in accordance with the published guidelines on perioperative anticoagulation. Relative contraindications include:

- Platelet count <100,000/ml
- APPT ratio or PT ratio >1.4

In these situations a decision to proceed to biopsy should be made following discussion with a hematologist.

"High-risk" patients should not have a biopsy performed as an outpatient procedure.

2.4 Type of Biopsies

There are guidelines and high-quality reviews for biopsy procedures [19–22]. Biopsies may be classified according to the type of access, such as percutaneous, bronchoscopic, laparoscopic, and open surgery biopsies, or to the tissue type of the sample obtained (cytological or histological). The type of tissue needed depends on the reason for biopsy, such as disease affecting an organ, like lung or liver, or type of lesion [23].

Percutaneous biopsies consist of two types: fine-needle aspiration (FNA) biopsy and cutting or core biopsy [19, 24]. Fine-needle aspiration needles are usually 20–25 gauge and provide suitable cells for cytological and microbiological examination. Core biopsy needles are usually larger disposable needles (18–20 gauge) with outer cannula (metal tube) and inner, notched rod in which a tissue specimen is cut, trapped, and withdrawn (Fig. 2.1). Core biopsies provide cores of tissue suitable for histological examination. Automated core needles are available and provide a more efficient and easier way to get the specimens (Fig. 2.2). The diagnostic accuracy of FNA is almost as good as core biopsy for the diagnosis of malignant lesions, especially if an onsite cytopathologist is

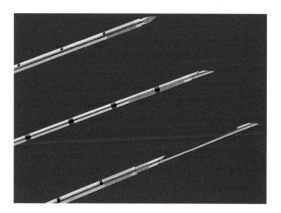

Fig. 2.1 Cutting or core biopsy needle in which a tissue specimen is cut, trapped, and withdrawn

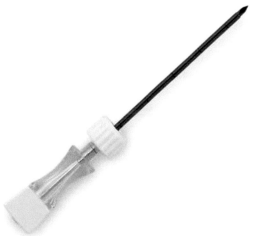

Fig. 2.3 Coaxial needle

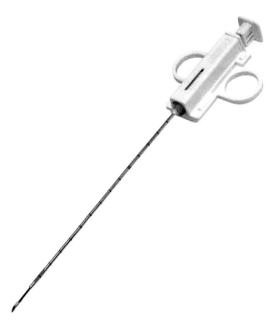

Fig. 2.2 Semi-automated core biopsy needle

present. However, for the diagnosis of benign lesions and lymphoma, core biopsy is preferred [2, 3, 25, 26].

Both FNA and core biopsies can be performed using a single needle or a coaxial technique. With the single needle technique, a needle is directly advanced into the lesion and multiple passes provide multiple samples. Alternatively, the coaxial technique involves the initial placement of a guiding needle at the edge of the target lesion, followed by the introduction of a thinner

biopsy needle through guiding needle to sample the lesion (Fig. 2.3). The disadvantage of the single needle technique is that positioning of the needle needs to be done with image guidance for each fragment to be collected, resulting in longer procedure time and a higher risk of complications. While a coaxial technique offers many advantages, the cost of the procedure is higher and a larger caliber guiding needle is required to make the path through the lesion. As an example, to perform a lung lesion biopsy, a larger needle will puncture the pleura. In the presence of a prominent air-bronchogram or open-bronchus sign in the lesion, a coaxial technique should be used more carefully as there is a higher risk of air embolism.

With the coaxial technique, a 17–19-gauge needle can be used as the guide, followed by insertion of a longer length 18- or 20-gauge needle [27]. In our institute, we use the coaxial biopsy set containing a 19-gauge guiding needle with a 20-gauge biopsy needle for obtaining tissue. The needle length should be selected depending on depth of lesion from the skin. In the core biopsy set available at our institution, the outer guiding needle is 2.5 cm shorter than the inner biopsy needle, and this is a very important point to be remembered during needle selection. Automated core biopsy needles are available with different lengths of specimen notch, such as 1.0 or 2.0 cm. Longer specimen notch is preferred as it provides longer cores of tissue; on the other hand, if the lesion is smaller than 1.0 cm, a short notch could be used to avoid injury to the normal structures.

The anticipated path of the needle is calculated on the CT console by extrapolating the path of the needle to the lesion. For the biopsy, a guiding needle is placed in the soft tissue and all necessary adjustments are done to align the needle with the target lesion prior to puncturing critical structures like pleura or peritoneum [1]. Especially for peripheral pulmonary lesions, the needle is advanced in one stroke into the lung until the edge of the lesion or at least 1–2 cm inside the lung. Leaving at least 1–2 cm needle inside the lung parenchyma avoids the needle slipping into the pleural space during respiratory motion and prevents laceration of the pleura by the needle tip. This is especially important when the lesion is located in lower and upper lung areas where the lesion moves significantly with breathing [1, 27]. After entry into lung, the needle should be left moving freely with respiration and should be touched only during breath hold.

Although reports show that there has been no correlation between the number of passes made and the incidence of pneumothorax [28], many authors have found that multiple punctures have been associated with a higher risk of pneumothorax and procedure failure [29]. To minimize complications, the pleura should be punctured only once [27]. The development of pneumothorax usually required abandoning the procedure, unless the lesion is stable and located close to the pleura [30].

Although rates for complications are similar for FNA and core biopsy needles, a slightly higher incidence of bleeding is reported with core biopsy needles [19]. There is little evidence in the literature that the needle caliber affects the complication rate within the size range of the smaller needles available for lung biopsy; bleeding and pneumothorax are more common with needles larger than 18 gauge [25, 27, 28].

2.5   PET/CT-Guided Biopsy: Procedure Description

Standard PET/CT images are acquired according to protocols described in national/international guidelines. ^{18}F-FDG PET/CT images are interpreted by imaging physicians with expertise in PET/CT imaging. After acquisition of the ^{18}F-FDG PET/CT images, the biopsy site and needle path are identified according to the location of the lesion and its relationship to anatomic structures.

Patients are positioned and immobilized according to the location of the lesion and the approach for the biopsy procedure. After completion of asepsis and antisepsis, local anesthesia is performed. Conscious sedation might be required when patients are anxious or noncooperative. The need for general anesthesia is uncommon.

If the coaxial technique is chosen, a suitable coaxial needle is inserted at the site previously identified. The angle and direction of the needle are adjusted according to the position of the suspicious lesion under the guidance of CT fluoroscopic imaging or CT acquisition. After placing the tip of the coaxial needle at the edge of the lesion, PET/CT images are acquired in one bed position to confirm and document the correct position of the coaxial needle.

The coaxial needle core is removed and a semiautomatic biopsy needle is inserted. The location of the needle is confirmed under fluoroscopy/CT scan and the biopsy site is imaged for documentation. If the lesion is small or difficult to be differentiated from important structures such as peripheral vessels, contrast-enhanced CT can be used for optimization of the images. Then, the specimens are cut and drawn at 1- or 2-cm fragments. Three or four specimens are collected. After needle removal, manual compression at the puncture site should be applied for 2–5 min. The specimens are fixed in 10 % formalin and sent for histopathological examination. Intraoperative histopathological examination with frozen sections is useful to reduce the need of performing repeat biopsies due to sampling error.

Patients are observed for at least 3 h after the procedure to ensure hemodynamic stability and monitoring the respiratory condition. CT is performed immediately and 3 h after the biopsy procedure in patients in whom the needle punctured the pleura, liver, or stomach wall during the biopsy procedure.

2.6   Types of Access

2.6.1   Direct Access

Direct access is usually used in soft tissue lesions. It is the simplest way to obtain a specimen (Figs. 2.4, 2.5, 2.6, and 2.7). For example, when a lesion is suspicious for sarcoma, the needle should be placed along the planned surgical access for resecting the lesion due to the possibility of tumor cell seeding along the needle tract. Although tumor cell seeding is uncommon and the relationship between biopsy and later recurrence is difficult to confirm, it is sometimes considered a major contraindication to certain biopsy procedures. Therefore, this potential complication of biopsy procedures needs to be discussed with the patient during the informed consent process [31–33]. Direct access is illustrated in Case 2.1, 2.2, 2.3, and 2.4.

2.6.2   Oblique Access

If a major vessel or a bone is along the way of a planned trajectory for the biopsy, various maneuvers can be helpful such as changing the position of the patient's leg or arm, taking a more medial or lateral path (Fig. 2.8), rotating the patient, puncturing the patient from the opposite side if feasible, and changing the respiration [34]. A lesion that cannot be accessed due to an intervening bone or vascular structure can also be approached using angled insertion of the biopsy needle in the craniocaudal axis (Fig. 2.8). While angling the CT gantry is not an option with PET/CT equipment, changing the craniocaudal angle of the needle is an option. Coronal and sagittal multiplanar CT reconstructions are very useful to determine the required angulation and the skin entry site. Oblique access is illustrated in Case 2.5.

2.6.3   Parasternal Approaches to the Mediastinal Lesions

The parasternal approach is used for the biopsy of anterior and middle mediastinal lesions when the lesion can be accessed from the lateral margin of the sternum [26]. With this approach, the needle is inserted directly into the target lesion or through the intervening fat (Fig. 2.9). The patient is usually placed in the supine position; occasionally, the lateral decubitus position may be helpful for creating a safe window. The internal mammary vessels should always be identified as they are located lateral to the sternal margin, and inadvertent injury may result in the formation of a hematoma. In most cases, a needle is inserted close to the lateral margin of the sternum and medial to these vessels. The degree of contact between the mediastinum and the parasternal chest wall may vary with breathing during the biopsy procedure, resulting in inadvertent puncture of the pleura or lung (Fig. 2.10). Parasternal access is illustrated in Cases 2.6 and 2.7.

2.6.4   Paravertebral Approach

The paravertebral approach is usually used for obtaining a biopsy from the retroperitoneum (Fig. 2.11) and from the middle and posterior mediastinal lesions. In the thorax, a needle is advanced through the space between the endothoracic fascia and parietal pleura (Fig. 2.12). The presence of the aorta makes this approach difficult from the left side. The patient is usually positioned in the prone or lateral decubitus position. In some patients, the space between the endothoracic fascia and parietal pleura is wide enough for direct advancement of the biopsy needle. Occasionally, this extrapleural space needs to be widened by injection of saline solution to create a window for needle entry (Fig. 2.12). Advancing the needle from the paravertebral approach without displacing the parietal pleura away from the spine may lead to inadvertent puncture of the pleura and lung. In addition, the paravertebral approach has the potential risk of injury to the esophagus, azygos vein, paravertebral vessels, intercostal vessels and nerves, as well as the spinal and vagus nerves.

Paravertebral access is illustrated in Cases 2.8 and 2.9.

2.6.5 Bone and Transbone Approach

Bone biopsy and transbone approach involves needle placement through the bone (Figs. 2.13 and 2.14) using the coaxial needle technique. In our experience, an 18-gauge guide needle is adequate to penetrate the sternum and to biopsy lytic lesions. For blastic lesions, 20-gauge or larger needles are recommended.

Transbone and bone needle insertion performed with local anesthesia and conscious sedation is well tolerated by patients. The administration of a local anesthetic on the periosteum minimizes the discomfort associated with the procedure. To avoid motion of the patient, it is important to place the patient in a comfortable position and minimize the time required to complete the biopsy. In the trans-sternal approach, intravenous administration of a contrast may be needed during the procedure to help identify the vascular structures.

Bone and transbone approach is illustrated in Cases 2.10 and 2.11.

2.6.6 Transpulmonary Approach to the Mediastinal Lesions

A transpulmonary path is used when a mediastinal lesion cannot be approached by the extrapleural route (Fig. 2.15) [25–27]. The patient is positioned according to the location of the lesion. Other precautions are similar to a lung biopsy. The coaxial needle passes through the lung parenchyma and two layers of visceral pleura.

2.6.7 Approach to Lung Lesion

Generally the shortest intercostal route is taken during lung biopsies, avoiding pulmonary fissures, bullous lesions, and emphysematous areas [27, 29]. Sometimes, pulmonary masses have associated collapsed or consolidated lung. ^{18}F-FDG PET/CT is helpful to differentiate malignant lesions that have usually intense uptake from associated inflammation and atelectasis that have moderate uptake (Figs. 2.16 and 2.17). It is preferable to access the lesion through a non-aerated route to avoid the risk of pneumothorax. When the lesion is cavitary or has air bronchogram, the biopsy is obtained from the wall of the lesion or the most solid part of the lesion (Fig. 2.18) [35].

2.7   ¹⁸F-FDG PET/CT-Guided Biopsy: Case Presentations

Case 2.1
History

This 64-year-old female presented with a history of treated leukemia and a mass in the subcutaneous tissues of the left cheek enlarging in the last 6 weeks. There was no response to antibiotic therapy.

¹⁸F-FDG PET/CT findings

The ¹⁸F-FDG PET/CT MIP (a) and axial images (d and e) showed intense uptake in the lesion measuring 41 mm in largest dimension on CT.

Biopsy procedure

The patient was positioned in the supine position with the head immobilized with traps. Direct access was the easiest and safest path to the lesion and chosen for core biopsy with 18G needle (b and c). Especially in soft tissue and bone lesions, the path of a future surgery should be considered in the definition of the biopsy access. The biopsy access should be removed in the surgery since epithelization of the biopsy path might occur.

Diagnosis

Histology and immunohistochemistry revealed poorly differentiated neuroendocrine tumor.

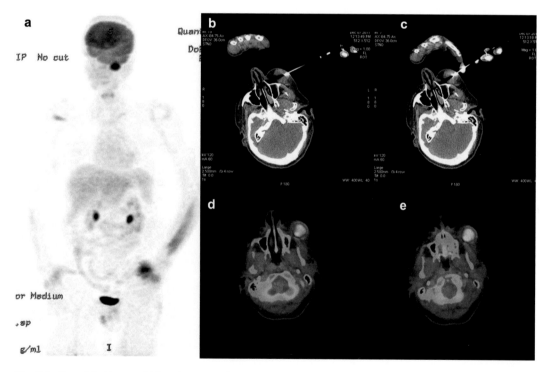

Fig. 2.4 Case 2.1. 64-year-old female presented with a history of treated leukemia and a mass in the subcutaneous tissues of the left cheek enlarging in the last 6 weeks

Case 2.2

This 52-year-old male presented with a history of weight loss, fever, and hip pain. Pelvis radiography revealed a large left iliac lytic lesion (not shown).

^{18}F-FDG PET/CT findings

^{18}F-FDG PET/CT MIP image (a) revealed multiple lymph nodes with intense ^{18}F-FDG uptake and bone lesions. Axial PET/CT images (d and e) shows large soft tissue extension of the lytic lesion.

Biopsy procedure

Biopsy was performed with direct access of soft tissue lesion with 18G needle (b and c).

Histology and immunohistochemistry revealed diffuse large B-cell lymphoma.

The patient was positioned in the prone position with pelvis immobilized. Direct access to the lesion with higher uptake was the easiest and safest path to the lesion and chosen for biopsy (b and c). A single bed position of ^{18}F-FDG PET/CT (d and e) was acquired to confirm needle position in an area within ^{18}F-FDG uptake.

Diagnosis

Histology and immunohistochemical analysis revealed diffuse large B-cell lymphoma.

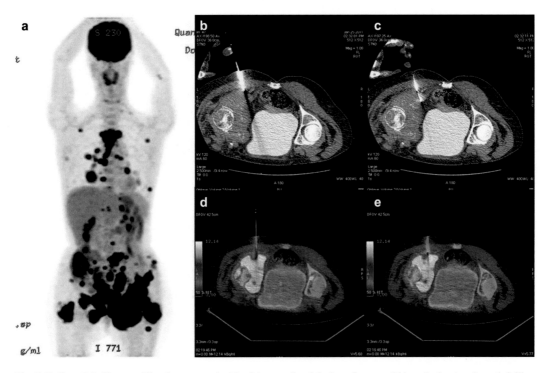

Fig. 2.5 Case 2.2. 52-year-old male presented with a history of weight loss, fever, and hip pain due to a large left iliac lytic lesion

Case 2.3

This 48-year-old male presented with a history of weight loss, hematuria, and abdominal pain. CT revealed a large right renal mass.

Biopsy was performed with direct access to the renal lesion (b and c).

18F-FDG PET/CT findings

18F-FDG PET/CT MIP (a) and axial PET/CT images (d and e) revealed heterogenous 18F-FDG uptake in the renal lesion measuring 146 mm in the largest diameter. There were also 18F-FDG -avid lymph nodes and a lung mass.

Biopsy procedure

The patient was positioned in the prone position. Direct intercostal access was the easiest path to the area of highest uptake in the lesion and chosen for biopsy (b and c) with an 18G needle.

Diagnosis

Histology and immunohistochemistry revealed renal cell carcinoma.

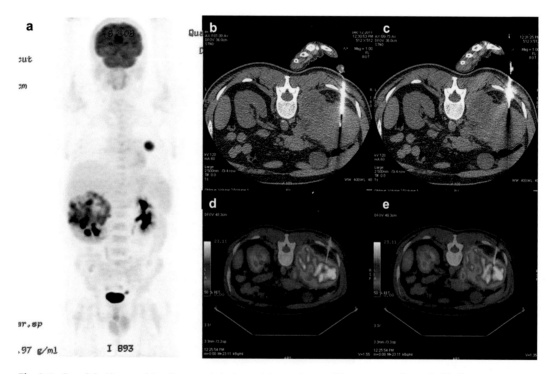

Fig. 2.6 Case 2.3. 48-year-old male presented a large right renal mass. Biopsy was performed with direct access to the renal lesion

Case 2.4

This 31-year-old male with a history of follicular lymphoma treated with chemotherapy and radiation therapy 2 years earlier presented with recurrence of B symptoms.

^{18}F-FDG PET/CT findings

The ^{18}F-FDG PET/CT MIP image (a) showed multiple ^{18}F-FDG-avid lymph nodes and hepatic, splenic, and bone marrow lesions. Axial PET/CT images (d and e) of the liver showed multiple lesions with ^{18}F-FDG uptake.

Biopsy procedure

The patient was positioned in the supine position with immobilization of the pelvis with arms above the head in a comfortable position. Direct access of a peripheral liver lesion was the easiest and safest path for biopsy (b and c) with an 18G needle.

Diagnosis

Histology and immunohistochemistry confirmed lymphoma recurrence.

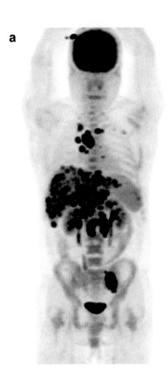
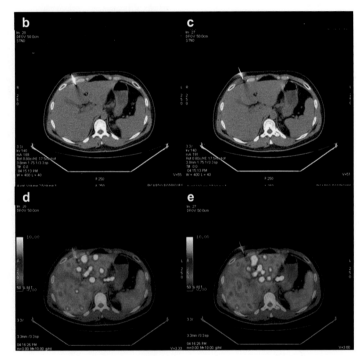

Fig. 2.7 Case 2.4. 31-year-old male with a history of follicular lymphoma treated with chemotherapy and radiation therapy 2 years earlier presented with recurrence of B symptoms

Case 2.5

This 68-year-old male presented with multiple pulmonary lesions.

^{18}F-FDG PET/CT findings

The ^{18}F-FDG PET/CT MIP image (a) showed a left pulmonary lesion centrally located, a left subpleural pulmonary lesion, and mediastinal lymph nodes with ^{18}F-FDG uptake. There was also focal ^{18}F-FDG uptake in the right colon. Axial PET/CT images (d and e) of the left subpleural lesion showed interposition of the scapula for direct access biopsy.

Biopsy procedure

The patient was positioned in the supine position with the head immobilized. The lung lesion was the most peripheral lesion and easier lesion to perform the biopsy. A direct access was planned to reach the lesion for biopsy; however, the scapula and costal arch blocked the direct access (d). Repositioning the arm of the patient did not free the direct access (b and c). The oblique access was chosen. Oblique puncture of the pleura increases the chance of pneumothorax, which did occur in this patient (c). During follow-up, the patient remained asymptomatic, and no chest tube was required.

Diagnosis

1. Histology revealed fungal infection.
2. Colonoscopy revealed an adenoma in the right colon.

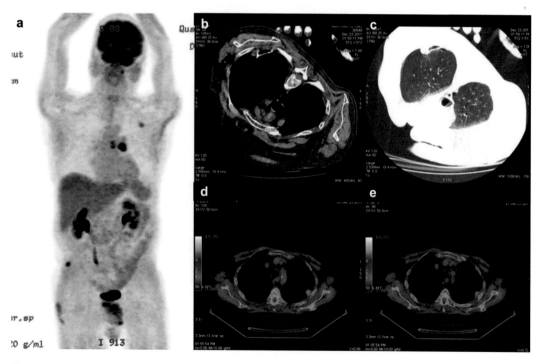

Fig. 2.8 Case 2.5. 68-year-old male presented with multiple pulmonary lesions

Case 2.6

This 68-year-old male presented with a mediastinal mass.

18F-FDG PET/CT findings

The ^{18}F-FDG PET/CT MIP image (a) showed mediastinal lymph nodes with ^{18}F-FDG uptake. The axial PET/CT images (d and e) showed a 39 mm anterior mediastinal lymph node.

Biopsy procedure

The patient was positioned in a supine comfortable position. Parasternal access was the easiest path to the lesion and chosen for biopsy (b and c). There was a small window between the mediastinal fat and the lesion. A saline solution was injected to enlarge the space for parasternal access biopsy (c and d). The internal mammary vessels were identified and an 18G needle was inserted medially to the mammary vessels.

Diagnosis

Histology and immunohistochemistry demonstrated classical Hodgkin lymphoma.

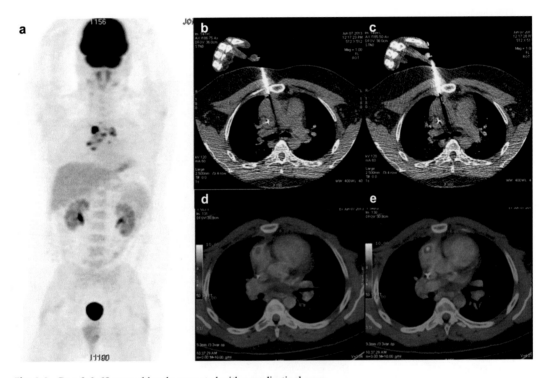

Fig. 2.9 Case 2.6. 68-year-old male presented with a mediastinal mass

Case 2.7

This 37-year-old male presented with right pulmonary nodules.

^{18}F-FDG PET/CT findings

The ^{18}F-FDG PET/CT MIP image (a) showed the lung nodules, pleural lesions, and mediastinal lymph nodes with intense ^{18}F-FDG uptake. The axial PET/CT images (d and e) showed the largest mediastinal lymph node selected for biopsy.

Biopsy procedure

The largest mediastinal lymph node was selected for biopsy as the safest lesion instead of the lung lesions. A parasternal access biopsy with an 18G core needle (b, c, and d) resulted in the inadvertent puncture of the right lung (b and c).

Diagnosis

Histology and immunohistochemistry demonstrated non-small cell lung cancer.

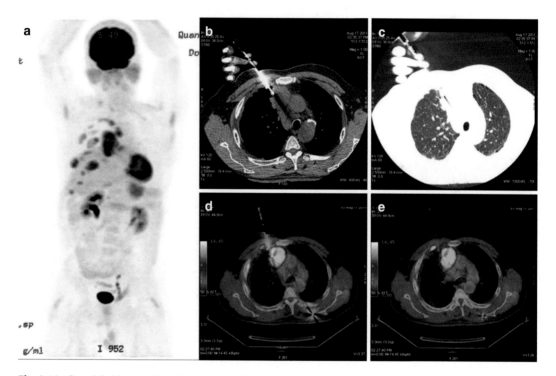

Fig. 2.10 Case 2.7. 37-year-old male presented with right pulmonary nodules

Case 2.8

This 50-year-old female presented with a retro-peritoneal mass.

18F-FDG PET/CT findings

The ^{18}F-FDG PET/CT MIP (a) and axial ^{18}F-FDG PET/CT (d and e) images showed the retroperitoneal mass with intense ^{18}F-FDG uptake suspicious for malignancy.

The ^{18}F-FDG PET/CT MIP (a) and axial images (d and e) showed intense uptake in the lesion measuring 127 mm in largest dimension on CT.

Biopsy procedure

The patient was positioned in the prone position. The paravertebral access was used to perform the biopsy (b and c) as anterior and lateral access would imply penetrating the liver.

Diagnosis

Histology and immunohistochemistry demonstrated poorly differentiated sarcoma.

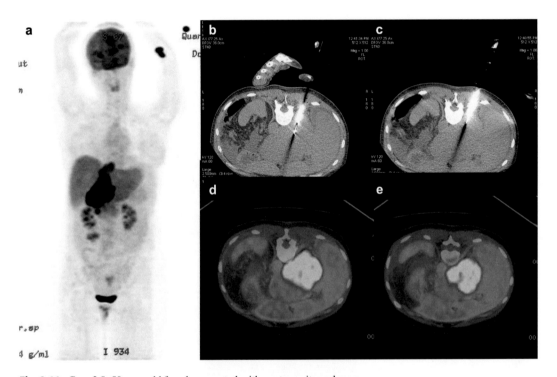

Fig. 2.11 Case 2.8. 50-year-old female presented with a retroperitoneal mass

Case 2.9

This 26-year-old female presented with shortness of breath and a large mediastinal mass.

^{18}F-FDG PET/CT findings

The ^{18}F-FDG PET/CT MIP (a) and axial images (d and f) showed the mediastinal mass with mild ^{18}F-FDG uptake. Axial CT image (e) and PET/CT image (f) showed that the left subclavian artery was precluding anterior access (cross lines).

Biopsy procedure

The anterior wall direct access was not possible due to the subclavian vessels (e and f). The paravertebral access was the alternate option; however, the extrapleural space was not large enough (e and f), and saline solution was injected to create a window for 18G needle entry (d and g).

Diagnosis

Histology and immunohistochemistry revealed a solitary fibrous tumor.

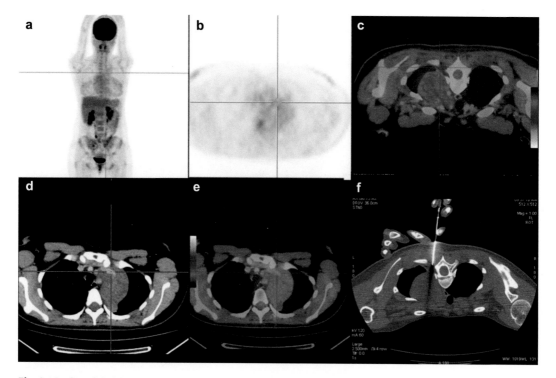

Fig. 2.12 Case 2.9. 26-year-old female presented with shortness of breath and a large mediastinal mass

Case 2.10

This 67-year-old female presented with hip pain. Pelvic radiography demonstrated a lytic lesion in the left iliac wing.

^{18}F-FDG PET/CT findings

The ^{18}F-FDG PET/CT MIP image (a) showed pulmonary lesions, mediastinal lymph nodes, and left iliac wing lesion with ^{18}F-FDG uptake. The axial PET/CT images (d and e) confirmed the ^{18}F-FDG uptake in the lung and mediastinal lymph nodes.

Biopsy procedure

The patient was positioned in the supine position with arms immobilized above the head. The biopsy of the mediastinal lymph nodes was chosen instead of lung biopsy, as lesions presented similar uptake and the lung lesions were not so peripheral (d and e). Direct access of the lymph nodes would require penetration through the lung. Trans-sternal access was used instead to perform the core biopsy of the mediastinal lymph nodes (b and c) with 18G needle.

Diagnosis

Histology and immunohistochemistry revealed lung adenocarcinoma.

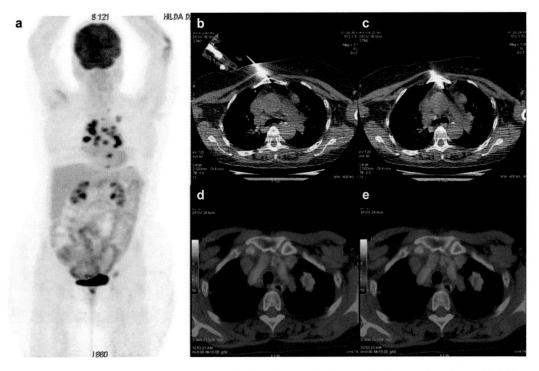

Fig. 2.13 Case 2.10. 67-year-old female presented with pulmonary lesions, mediastinal lymph nodes, and left iliac wing lesion

Case 2.11

This 60-year-old male presented with a left pulmonary mass.

¹⁸F-FDG PET/CT findings

The ¹⁸F-FDG PET/CT MIP image (a) showed pulmonary lesions, mediastinal lymph nodes, and multiple bone lesions with intense ¹⁸F-FDG uptake. The axial PET/CT images (d and e) confirmed the ¹⁸F-FDG uptake in a lytic lesion in the sacrum.

Biopsy procedure

In a patient with multiple lung, lymph node, and bone lesions, choosing a representative lesion for biopsy takes into account the ¹⁸F-FDG uptake and the risk of complications of the procedure. As a bone biopsy presents lower than lung biopsy, a bone biopsy technique was used to perform the sacrum biopsy with an 18G needle (b and c).

Diagnosis

Histology and immunohistochemistry revealed lung adenocarcinoma.

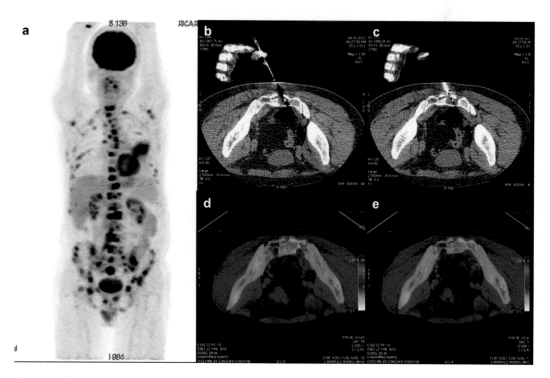

Fig. 2.14 Case 2.11. 60-year-old male presented with a left pulmonary mass

Case 2.12

A 50-year-old male with a prior history of melanoma and surgery 4 years ago presented with a posterior mediastinal mass.

18F-FDG PET/CT findings

The 18F-FDG PET/CT MIP image (a) showed the mediastinal mass with 18F-FDG uptake.

Biopsy procedure

The axial PET/CT images (d and e) of the posterior mediastinal mass showed no window for direct access of the mass. A posterior transpulmonary access was used to perform the biopsy (c and d) as the anterior access was not possible due to the presence of the heart and major vessels. The coaxial needle technique was chosen as it has a lower risk of seeding neoplastic cells in the punctured lung than a non-coaxial technique.

Diagnosis

Histology and immunohistochemical analysis confirmed melanoma recurrence.

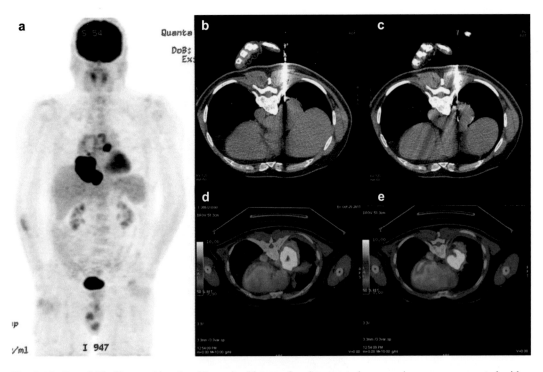

Fig. 2.15 Case 2.12. 50-year-old male with a prior history of melanoma and surgery 4 years ago presented with a posterior mediastinal mass

Case 2.13

This 77-year-old male presented with a necrotic mass in the right lung.

^{18}F-FDG PET/CT findings

The ^{18}F-FDG PET/CT MIP image (a) showed intense uptake in the pulmonary mass but also in a large hepatic mass. The axial PET/CT images (d and e) of the pulmonary mass showed uptake in the periphery of the mass and central necrosis.

As the lung mass was peripheral, the lung mass was chosen as target for biopsy.

Biopsy procedure

Direct pulmonary access was used to perform the biopsy (b and c) taking into account the region with higher ^{18}F-FDG uptake (c and d).

Diagnosis

Histology and immunohistochemistry revealed poorly differentiated carcinoma.

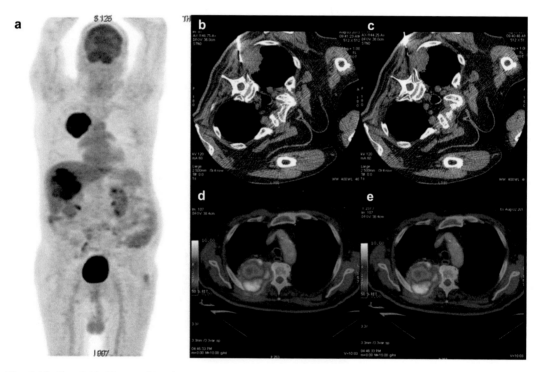

Fig. 2.16 Case 2.13. 77-year-old male presented with a necrotic mass in the right lung

Case 2.14

This 50-year-old female presented with a large pulmonary heterogenous mass.

18F-FDG PET/CT findings

The 18F-FDG PET/CT MIP image (a) showed heterogenous uptake in the large mass of the left lung. Additional 18F-FDG-avid lymph nodes and contralateral pulmonary lesions are seen. The axial PET/CT images (d and e) of the left pulmonary mass showed intense uptake in the solid portion of the mass and mild to moderate uptake in the adjacent atelectasis.

Biopsy procedure

Direct pulmonary access was best to perform the biopsy of the portion of the mass with highest 18F-FDG uptake identified on the 18F-FDG PET images (c and d).

Diagnosis

Histology and immunohistochemistry revealed adenocarcinoma.

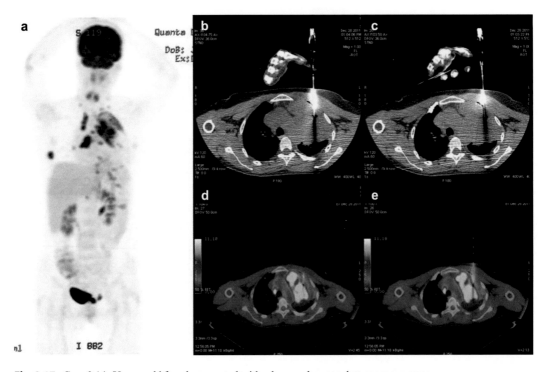

Fig. 2.17 Case 2.14. 50-year-old female presented with a large pulmonary heterogenous mass

Case 2.15

This 73-year-old female presented with lung consolidation of the right lower lobe. The patient was treated with antibiotics without success. The area of consolation enlarged on a follow-up CT.

¹⁸F-FDG PET/CT findings

The ¹⁸F-FDG PET/CT MIP image (a) showed moderate ¹⁸F-FDG uptake in the area of consolidation. The axial PET/CT images (d and e) showed ¹⁸F-FDG uptake mainly in the periphery of the lesion and the presence of air bronchogram.

Biopsy procedure

Direct pulmonary access was best to perform the biopsy of the portion of the consolidation with the highest ¹⁸F-FDG uptake identified on the ¹⁸F-FDG PET images (c and d). When the lesion has air bronchogram, the biopsy is obtained from the most solid part of the lesion, trying to avoid bronchogram due to the higher risk of hemoptysis.

Diagnosis

Histology and immunohistochemistry revealed adenocarcinoma with predominant lepidic growth pattern (previous classified as bronchioalveolar carcinoma).

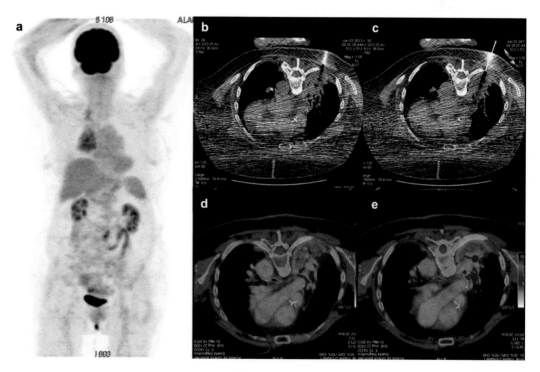

Fig. 2.18 Case 2.15. 73-year-old female presented with lung consolidation of the right lower lobe. The patient was treated with antibiotics without success. The area of consolation enlarged on a follow-up CT

References

1. Cerci JJ, Pereira Neto CC, Krauzer C, Sakamoto DG, Vitola JV. The impact of coaxial core biopsy guided by FDG PET/CT in oncological patients. Eur J Nucl Med Mol Imaging. 2013;40(1):98–103.

2. Purandare NC, Kulkarni AV, Kulkarni SS, Roy D, Agrawal A, Shah S, Rangarajan V. 18F-FDG PET/CT-directed biopsy: does it offer incremental benefit? Nucl Med Commun. 2013;34(3):203–10.

3. O'Sullivan PJ, Rohren EM, Madewell JE. Positron emission tomography-CT imaging in guiding musculoskeletal biopsy. Radiol Clin North Am. 2008;46(3):475–86.

4. Govindarajan MJ, Nagaraj KR, Kallur KG, Sridhar PS. PET/CT guidance for percutaneous fine needle aspiration cytology/biopsy. Indian J Radiol Imaging. 2009;19:208–9. PubMed: 19881087.

5. Tatli S, Gerbaudo VH, Mamede M, Tuncali K, Shyn PB, Silverman SG. Abdominal masses sampled at PET/CT-guided percutaneous biopsy: initial experience with registration of prior PET/CT images. Radiology. 2010;256(1):305–11.

6. Klaeser B, Wiskirchen J, Wartenberg J, Weitzel T, Schmid RA, Mueller MD, Krause T. PET/CT-guided biopsies of metabolically active bone lesions: applications and clinical impact. Eur J Nucl Med Mol Imaging. 2010;37(11):2027–36.

7. Werner MK, Aschoff P, Reimold M, Pfannenberg C. FDG-PET/CT-guided biopsy of bone metastases sets a new course in patient management after extensive imaging and multiple futile biopsies. Br J Radiol. 2011;84(999):e65–7.

8. Venkatesan AM, Kadoury S, Abi-Jaoudeh N, Levy EB, Maass-Moreno R, Krücker J, Dalal S, Xu S, Glossop N, Wood BJ. Real-time FDG PET guidance during biopsies and radiofrequency ablation using multimodality fusion with electromagnetic navigation. Radiology. 2011;260(3):848–56.

9. Win AZ, Aparici CM. Real-time FDG PET/CT-guided bone biopsy in a patient with two primary malignancies. Eur J Nucl Med Mol Imaging. 2013;40(11):1787–8.

10. Fukuda H, Kubota K, Matsuzawa T. Pioneering and fundamental achievements on the development of positron emission tomography (PET) in oncology. Tohoku J Exp Med. 2013;230(3):155–69. PubMed PMID: 23883588.

11. Stewart FW. The diagnosis of tumors by aspiration. Am J Pathol. 1933;9:801–12.

12. Slomka PJ. Software approach to merging molecular with anatomic information. J Nucl Med. 2004;45 Suppl 1:36S–45.

13. Massager N, David P, Goldman S, et al. Combined magnetic resonance imaging and positron emission tomography-guided stereotactic biopsy in brainstem mass lesions: diagnostic yield in a series of 30 patients. J Neurosurg. 2000;93(6):951–7.

14. Maintz JB, Viergever MA. A survey of medical image registration. Med Image Anal. 1998;2(1):1–36.

15. Shekhar R, Walimbe V, Raja S, et al. Automated 3-dimensional elastic registration of whole-body PET and CT from separate or combined scanners. J Nucl Med. 2005;46(9):1488–96.

16. Lindblom K. Diagnostic kidney puncture in cysts and tumors. AJR. 1952;68:209–15.

17. Brix G, Lechel U, Glatting G, et al. Radiation exposure of patients undergoing whole-body dual-modality 18 F-FDG PET/CT examinations. J Nucl Med. 2005;46:608–13.

18. Solbiati L, Cova L, Terace T, Zaid S. Realtime, ultrasound-CT/MRI fusion imaging for planning, guiding, and immediately assessing percutaneous radiofrequency ablation of liver malignancies: analysis of results in 225 patients and 426 tumors (abstr). In: Radiological Society of North America scientific assembly and annual meeting program. Oak Brook: Radiological Society of North America; 2008. p. 552.

19. Manhire A, Charig M, Clelland C, Gleeson F, Miller R, Moss H, Pointon K, Richardson C, Sawicka E. BTS. Guidelines for radiologically guided lung biopsy. Thorax. 2003;58(11):920–36. PubMed PMID: 14586042.

20. Gogna A, Peh WC, Munk PL. Image-guided musculoskeletal biopsy. Radiol Clin North Am. 2008;46(3):455–73.

21. Uppot RN, Harisinghani MG, Gervais DA. Imaging-guided percutaneous renal biopsy: rationale and approach. AJR Am J Roentgenol. 2010;194(6):1443–9.

22. Chuah SY. Liver biopsy–past, present and future. Singapore Med J. 1996;37(1):86–90.

23. Lal H, Neyaz Z, Nath A, Borah S. CT-guided percutaneous biopsy of intrathoracic lesions. Korean J Radiol. 2012;13(2):210–26.

24. Cham MD, Lane ME, Henschke CI, Yankelevitz DF. Lung biopsy: special techniques. Semin Respir Crit Care Med. 2008;29:335–49.

25. Klein JS, Salomon G, Stewart EA. Transthoracic needle biopsy with a coaxially placed 20-gauge automated cutting needle: results in 122 patients. Radiology. 1996;198:715–20.

26. Gupta S, Seaberg K, Wallace MJ, Madoff DC, Morello Jr FA, Ahrar K, et al. Imaging-guided percutaneous biopsy of mediastinal lesions: different approaches and anatomic considerations. Radiographics. 2005;25:763–88.

27. Moore EH. Technical aspects of needle aspiration lung biopsy: a personal perspective. Radiology. 1998;208:303–18.

28. Cox JE, Chiles C, McManus CM, Aquino SL, Choplin RH. Transthoracic needle aspiration biopsy: variables that affect risk of pneumothorax. Radiology. 1999;212:165–8.

29. Wallace AB, Suh RD. Percutaneous transthoracic needle biopsy: special considerations and techniques

used in lung transplant recipients. Semin Intervent Radiol. 2004;21:247–58.

30. Tsai IC, Tsai WL, Chen MC, Chang GC, Tzeng WS, Chan SW, et al. CT-guided core biopsy of lung lesions: a primer. AJR Am J Roentgenol. 2009;193:1228–35.

31. Robertson EG, Baxter G. Tumour seeding following percutaneous needle biopsy: the real story! Clin Radiol. 2011;66(11):1007–14.

32. Loughran CF, Keeling CR. Seeding of tumour cells following breast biopsy: a literature review. Br J Radiol. 2011;84(1006):869–74.

33. Silva MA, Hegab B, Hyde C, Guo B, Buckels JA, Mirza DF. Needle track seeding following biopsy of liver lesions in the diagnosis of hepatocellular cancer: a systematic review and meta-analysis. Gut. 2008;57(11):1592–6.

34. Blady JV. Aspiration biopsy of tumors in obscure or difficult locations under roentgenoscopic guidance. AJR. 1939;42:515–24.

35. Bandoh S, Fujita J, Fukunaga Y, Yokota K, Ueda Y, Okada H, et al. Cavitary lung cancer with an aspergilloma-like shadow. Lung Cancer. 1999;26: 195–8.

Acute Complications of Biopsy Procedures

3

Juliano J. Cerci, Mateos Bogoni,
and Dominique Delbeke

3.1   Introduction

Physicians should be able to identify and appro-
priately manage the complications of biopsy procedures. Resuscitation facilities and chest drain
equipment should be immediately available.
When a complication has occurred, the heart rate,
blood pressure, and oxygen saturation should be
monitored and recorded. Percutaneous biopsies
can be performed safely on an outpatient basis.
However, high-risk patients should not have a
biopsy performed as outpatient. A post-biopsy
image (supine chest radiograph, CT of the region
of concern) should be performed at least 1 h after
the procedure to assess the presence of pneumothorax or other complications. During the
informed consent process, patients should be
made aware of potential delayed complications
and given verbal and written instructions to return
if they become symptomatic. When biopsies are

performed on an outpatient basis, patients should
live within 30 min of a hospital, have adequate
home support, and have access to a telephone.

Physicians should audit their own practice at
least annually for complication rates to inform
patients before consent is given. False positives
should be less than 1 %, adequacy of sample
should be over 90 %, and sensitivity for malignancy should be within the range of 85–90 % for
lesions larger than 2 cm. The complication rate
should be similar to or better than those from the
literature: for example, for biopsy of the lungs,
the complication of pneumothorax should be less
than 20.5 % of biopsies, pneumothorax requiring
placement of a chest tube less than 3.1 %, hemoptysis less than 5.3 %, and death rate less than
0.15 % [1]. Early detection of complications and
timely management are important. Pneumothorax,
hemorrhage, hemothorax, and hematoma are the
most common complications [2–5]. Other less
common complications are vasovagal reaction,
hemomediastinum, cardiac tamponade, air embolism, and tumor seeding [1–5].

The incidence of post-biopsy pneumothorax
ranges from 27 to 54 % in most of the published
large series (Figs. 3.1 and 3.2), depending on the
type of follow-up modality (CT vs chest radiography vs clinical symptoms). Although most of these
cases can be managed conservatively, about 3–15 %
of patients require placement of a chest tube when
the pneumothorax becomes symptomatic or contin-
ues to increase in size [6–8]. In our experience, the

J.J. Cerci (✉)
Quanta – Diagnóstico e Terapia, Curitiba, PR, Brazil
e-mail: cercijuliano@hotmail.com

M. Bogoni
Hospital de Clínicas – Universidade Federal do
Paraná, Curitiba, PR, Brazil
e-mail: bogonimateos@gmail.com

D. Delbeke
Radiology and Radiological Sciences, Vanderbilt
University Medical Center, Nashville, TN, USA
e-mail: dominique.delbeke@vanderbilt.edu

© Springer International Publishing 2016
J. Cerci et al. (eds.), *Oncological PET/CT with Histological Confirmation*,
DOI 10.1007/978-3-319-27880-3_3

majority of pneumothorax are small and stable, and less than 1 % of the cases require intervention [9].

Pulmonary hemorrhage may occur with or without hemoptysis. While hemorrhage occurs in 5.0–16.9 % of the cases, it presents as hemoptysis in only 1.2–5.0 % of the patients [1]. If hemoptysis occurs, patients should be reassured and placed in the decubitus position with biopsy side down to prevent aspiration of blood in other areas of the lung (Fig. 3.3) [1, 5]. In most cases, hemoptysis is self-limiting and resolves with conservative treatment; however, massive hemoptysis is the most dreadful complication of a lung biopsy and should be promptly treated. The risk of pulmonary hemorrhage is higher in patients with vascular tumors, centrally located lesions, pulmonary hypertension, abnormal coagulation profile, and chronic inflammatory cavities due to the presence of hypertrophied bronchial arteries [1]. For patients with vascular lesions and bleeding disorders, small caliber needles should be used to reduce the risk of severe hemorrhage [1]. Pulmonary hemorrhage is also more common with the use of core biopsy needles.

Significant hematoma and hemothorax are rare but may develop if the intercostal or internal mammary arteries are injured during the biopsy procedure (Fig. 3.4). Pneumorrhachis, the

presence of intraspinal air, has been rarely reported after anesthetic interventions [10].

Air embolism is a very rare complication and it may affect the cerebral or coronary circulation [11]. The most likely etiology for air embolism is the introduction of ambient air into the pulmonary vein via the biopsy needle or the formation of a bronchovenous fistula along the needle path or in the biopsy cavity. Factors associated with air embolisms are coughing during the procedure, biopsy of consolidated lung, cavitary or cystic lesions, associated vasculitis, and use of the coaxial technique [8]. To prevent air embolism, the guiding needle should never be left without the inner stylet. During exchange of inner stylet with the biopsy needle, the hub of the guiding needle should be covered with the finger or thumb [8].

Other complications like tumor seeding along the needle tract [12–15], cardiac tamponade [16], and pneumonia/empyema [9] are extremely rare.

3.2   Case Presentations

Case 3.1
This 67-year-old male with previously treated colon cancer presented with pulmonary nodules on follow-up CT imaging 2 years later.

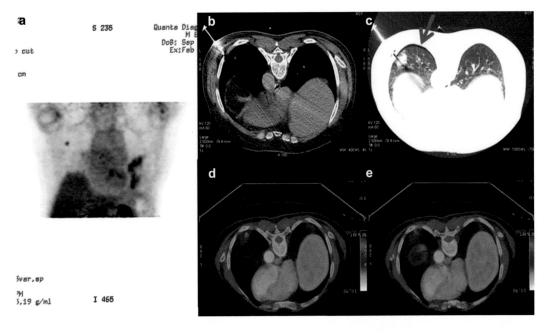

Fig. 3.1 Small pneumothorax (*arrow*) and hemorrhage following a lung biopsy of LLL lesion

^{18}F-FDG PET/CT findings

The ^{18}F-FDG PET/CT MIP (a) showed intense uptake in the lung lesions; axial ^{18}F-FDG PET/CT images (d and e) showed a left lower lobe (LLL) lesion measuring 12 mm in largest dimension on CT.

Biopsy procedure

The patient was positioned in the prone position with the arms immobilized in a comfortable position. Direct access was the easiest path to the lesion and chosen for biopsy (b and c). A small pneumothorax and hemorrhage occurred during the biopsy procedure (c). During follow-up, the patient remained asymptomatic, a follow-up CT showed the pneumothorax to be stable, and the patient was discharged 3 h later.

Diagnosis

Histology and immunohistochemistry demonstrated adenocarcinoma consistent with a colon primary metastatic to the lungs.

Case 3.2

This 36-year-old female with history treated breast cancer presented with a new left pulmonary nodule on follow-up imaging.

^{18}F-FDG PET/CT findings

The ^{18}F-FDG PET/CT MIP (a) showed intense uptake in the left apical lung lesion measuring 24 mm in largest dimension on CT.

Biopsy procedure

The patient was positioned in the prone position with the arms immobilized in a comfortable position. The posterior direct pulmonary access was best to perform the biopsy (b and c) due to the interposition of subclavian artery for the anterior shorter approach. A small pulmonary hemorrhage occurred following the biopsy. During follow-up, the 2 h chest radiography revealed a pneumothorax (arrow figures d and e). Although the pneumothorax was stable on follow-up imaging (e), the patient was hospitalized and monitored. The patient did not need placement of a chest tube and was discharged 2 days later.

Diagnosis

Histology and immunohistochemistry revealed adenocarcinoma, compatible with a primary breast cancer metastatic to the lungs.

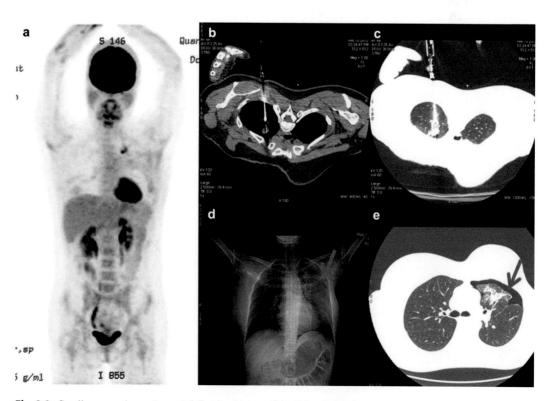

Fig. 3.2 Small pneumothorax (*arrow*) following biopsy of the left apical lesion

Case 3.3

This 73-year-old female with a history of lung cancer treated with surgery and radiotherapy presented with consolidation of the right lung. She was treated with antibiotics but the area of consolidation was increasing on follow-up imaging (not shown).

^{18}F-FDG PET/CT findings

The ^{18}F-FDG PET/CT MIP image (a) and axial images (c and d) showed moderate uptake in the area of consolidation, the presence of air bronchogram, and the cavitary lesions (arrow) in the right lower lobe (RLL).

Biopsy procedure

The patient was positioned in the prone position with the arms immobilized in a comfortable position. Direct pulmonary access was best to perform the biopsy of the portion of the consolidation with highest ^{18}F-FDG uptake identified on the ^{18}F-FDG PET images (a–d). The area of air bronchogram and cavitary lesion should be avoided (c and d). Even if the areas of air bronchogram and cavitary lesion were avoided, the

patient developed massive hemoptysis requiring intubation and blood transfusion.

Diagnosis

Histology and immunohistochemistry revealed lung cancer recurrence.

Case 3.4

This 34-year-old male with history of seminoma presented with new pulmonary nodules.

^{18}F-FDG PET/CT findings

The CT axial images (d and e) showed the left lower lobe (LLL) lesion measuring 8 mm in largest dimension on CT. The ^{18}F-FDG PET/CT axial PET/CT images (not shown) showed mild ^{18}F-FDG in the small nodules. The uptake was likely underestimated due to partial volume averaging is nodules below PET resolution. The larger nodule 8 mm and was located in the left lower lobe.

Biopsy procedure

The patient was positioned in the supine position with the arms immobilized in a comfortable position. Direct pulmonary access was best to

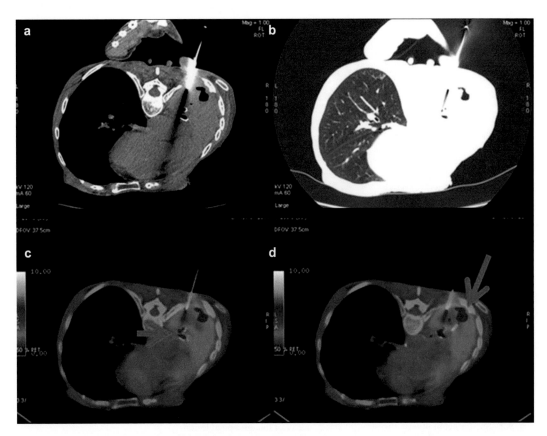

Fig. 3.3 Cavitary lesion and air bronchogram (*arrow*) in the RLL

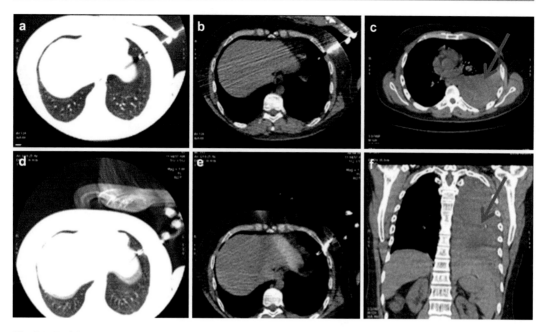

Fig. 3.4 Left hemothorax (*arrow*) following biopsy of the LLL lesion

perform the biopsy of the larger nodule (a, b, d and e). Patient developed a hemothorax (arrow figures c and f) requiring surgery and blood transfusion.

Diagnosis

Histology revealed tuberculosis.

References

1. Manhire A, Charig M, Clelland C, Gleeson F, Miller R, Moss H, et al. Guidelines for radiologically guided lung biopsy. Thorax. 2003;58:920–36.
2. Diamantis A, Magiorkinis E, Koutselini H. Fine-needle aspiration (FNA) biopsy: historical aspects. Folia Histochem Cytobiol. 2009;47(2):191–7.
3. Hopper KD. Percutaneous, radiographically guided biopsy: a history. Radiology. 1995;196:329–33.
4. Collings CL, Westcott JL, Banson NL, Lange RC. Pneumothorax and dependent versus nondependent patient position after needle biopsy of the lung. Radiology. 1999;210:59–64.
5. Wu CC, Maher MM, Shepard JA. Complications of CT-guided percutaneous needle biopsy of the chest: prevention and management. AJR. 2011;196:W678–82.
6. Moore EH. Technical aspects of needle aspiration lung biopsy: a personal perspective. Radiology. 1998; 208:303–18.
7. Cox JE, Chiles C, McManus CM, Aquino SL, Choplin RH. Transthoracic needle aspiration biopsy: variables that affect risk of pneumothorax. Radiology. 1999; 212:165–8.
8. Tsai IC, Tsai WL, Chen MC, Chang GC, Tzeng WS, Chan SW, et al. CT-guided core biopsy of lung lesions: a primer. AJR Am J Roentgenol. 2009;193:1228–35.
9. Cerci JJ, Pereira Neto CC, Krauzer C, Sakamoto DG, Vitola JV. The impact of coaxial core biopsy guided by FDG PET/CT in oncological patients. Eur J Nucl Med Mol Imaging. 2013;40(1):98–103.
10. Oertel MF, Korinth MC, Reinges MH, Krings T, Terbeck S, Gilsbach JM. Pathogenesis, diagnosis and management of pneumorrhachis. Eur Spine J. 2006;15 Suppl 5:636–43.
11. Hare SS, Gupta A, Goncalves AT, Souza CA, Matzinger F, Seely JM. Systemic arterial air embolism after percutaneous lung biopsy. Clin Radiol. 2011;66:589–96.
12. Sinner WN. Complications of percutaneous transthoracic needle aspiration biopsy. Acta Radiol Diagn (Stockh). 1976;17:813–28.
13. Silva MA, Hegab B, Hyde C, Guo B, Buckels JA, Mirza DF. Needle track seeding following biopsy of liver lesions in the diagnosis of hepatocellular cancer: a systematic review and meta-analysis. Gut. 2008; 57(11):1592–6. doi:10.1136/gut.2008.149062.
14. Loughran CF, Keeling CR. Seeding of tumour cells following breast biopsy: a literature review. Br J Radiol. 2011;84(1006):869–74. doi:10.1259/bjr/77245199. PubMed PMID: 21933978, Review.
15. Robertson EG, Baxter G. Tumour seeding following percutaneous needle biopsy: the real story! Clin Radiol. 2011;66(11):1007–14. doi:10.1016/j.crad.2011.05.012.
16. Kucharczyk W, Weisbrod GL, Cooper JD, Todd T. Cardiac tamponade as a complication of thin-needle aspiration lung biopsy. Chest. 1982;82(1): 120–1.

18F-FDG PET/CT for Guiding Biopsy in Lymphoma Patients

4

Francisca Redondo Moneta and Monica Celli

4.1 Introduction

The 2008 WHO clinicopathologic classification of lymphoid malignancies recognizes more than 30 subtypes of non-Hodgkin lymphomas (NHL), of which 85 % have a B-cell origin and 15 % derive from T cells. Hodgkin disease (HD) includes two entities, classical HD (95 %) and nodular lympho-cyte predominant Hodgkin lymphoma (5 %). Classical HD is further classified in four subtypes: nodular sclerosis, mixed cellularity, lymphocyte rich, and lymphocyte depletion [1].

The initial diagnosis of lymphoma is preferentially made by excisional node biopsy or, alternatively, core-needle biopsy from deep-seated nodal and extranodal sites of involvement. These techniques provide enough material for diagnosis of lymphoma subtypes using a combination of immunoarchitecture, immunophenotype, and molecular features [2–7]. The identification of specific molecular signatures may be required for diagnostic verification, prognostic stratification, and choice of appropriate therapy [8–12].

F.R. Moneta (✉)
Oncological Clinic Fundación Arturo López Pérez, Santiago, Chile
e-mail: fredondom@gmail.com

M. Celli
Ospedale Policlinico S.Orsola-Malpighi, Bologna, Italy
e-mail: moki.celli@gmail.com

With regard to B-cell NHL diagnosis, fine-needle aspiration (FNA) has become an option since immunophenotyping with multiparameter flow cytometry and ancillary tests has become available, avoiding the need for more invasive surgical procedures [13].

The clinical course of the disease, aggressive or indolent, is determined by the histological type of lymphoma and the stage at presentation [14]. Among the aggressive histological types, diffuse large B-cell lymphoma (DLBCL) accounts for nearly 30 % of adult NHL, generally arising ex novo or, less frequently, as the result of transformed low-grade lymphoma. Extranodal involvement at presentation is common (40 % of cases). When involved, bone marrow can be infiltrated by concordant high-grade disease or a discordant low-grade B-cell population. Burkitt lymphoma (BL) is a very aggressive B-cell malignancy accounting for 2 % of adult NHL and about 40 % of childhood lymphomas. Given its short doubling time, Burkitt lymphoma often presents with a bulky mass (abdominal masses are often associated with the sporadic variant of BL). Extranodal involvement is more common in children than adults [1].

Aggressive T-cell NHL comprise adult T-cell lymphoma, peripheral T-cell lymphoma, anaplastic large cell lymphoma (ALCL), and T lymphoblastic lymphoma.

Mantle cell lymphoma (MCL) is a rare B-cell lymphoma accounting for 5–10 % of NHL, often

© Springer International Publishing 2016
J. Cerci et al. (eds.), *Oncological PET/CT with Histological Confirmation*,
DOI 10.1007/978-3-319-27880-3_4

affecting individuals over the age of 60. Aggressive (i.e., blastoid and pleomorphic) and indolent (i.e., small-cell and marginal zone-like) variants have been reported. Advanced stage disease with lymphadenopathy, hepatosplenomegaly, and bone marrow infiltration is common at presentation [1].

Among indolent NHL, follicular lymphoma (FL) is the most common histological type accounting for 20 % of all adult NHL. Patients generally present with widespread disease, mainly involving the lymph nodes, spleen, and bone marrow. Histological grading refers to the proportion of observed centroblasts (i.e., large cells) in ten neoplastic follicles expressed per high-power fields (hpf). Follicular lymphomas graded 1 or 2 (less than 15 centroblasts/hpf) are clinically indolent, whereas grade 3 (more than 15 centroblasts/hpf) lymphomas behave in a more aggressive fashion. Grade 3B FL is often accompanied by areas of diffuse large B-cell lymphoma (70 % of grade 3B FL) [1].

Marginal zone lymphomas (MZL) are slow-growing B-cell malignancies, mainly occurring in adults over the age of 60, and account for 10 % of all NHL. Three subtypes can be recognized (nodal, extranodal, and splenic) being the extranodal marginal zone subtype or mucosa-associated lymphoid tissue (MALT) the most commonly encountered and the stomach the most affected organ. MALT lymphomas often arise on a chronic inflammatory background (e.g., *Helicobacter pylori* in gastric MALT) [1].

Aggressive lymphomas are considered potentially curable, whereas advanced indolent entities, although slow-growing, eventually progress.

In newly diagnosed lymphoma patients, ^{18}F-FDG PET/CT imaging is recommended for accurate staging of both nodal and extranodal involvement (Ann Arbor status), treatment planning, and prognostication [15–17]. Baseline ^{18}F-FDG PET/CT imaging also offers a basis for comparison to assess metabolic response during and after therapy [18].

Despite ^{18}F-FDG PET/CT undisputed superiority in staging most lymphomatous subtypes, mainly aggressive NHL and HD, ^{18}F-FDG uptake

has proved to vary among different histological types and within the same categories [19–21]. Aggressive NHL such as diffuse large B-cell lymphoma, Burkitt lymphoma, large cell anaplastic lymphoma, natural killer/T-cell lymphoma, lymphoblastic lymphoma, peripheral T-cell lymphoma, and nodular sclerosis-type HD usually exhibit very high ^{18}F-FDG avidity. Variable moderate-to-high ^{18}F-FDG uptake is seen in grade 3 follicular lymphoma, mantle cell lymphoma, adult T-cell lymphoma, and the mixed cellularity and lymphocyte depletion variants of classical HD. Indolent histotypes such as low-grade follicular lymphoma, marginal zone lymphoma (splenic or MALT associated), small lymphocytic lymphoma, and also lymphocyte predominant HD may show very low or absent ^{18}F-FDG uptake thus reducing ^{18}F-FDG PET/CT staging accuracy.

Despite a relatively low ^{18}F-FDG avidity, treatment-naive indolent lymphomas may still require a baseline ^{18}F-FDG PET/CT in order to rule out unexpected lesions in patients amenable to local treatment [22, 23]; to allow a wait-and-see strategy; to pinpoint lesions with unexpected high ^{18}F-FDG uptake, suspicious for histological transformation [24, 25]; and to identify sites of extranodal involvement otherwise difficult to evaluate on CT. It must be noted that ^{18}F-FDG PET/CT positivity is not lymphoma specific as other malignant and nonmalignant processes may mimic lymphoma (e.g., infections and chronic granulomatous diseases) [26] and that ^{18}F-FDG PET/CT accuracy in identifying extranodal lymphomatous disease can be negatively affected in organs with variable physiological ^{18}F-FDG activity. For instance, MALT marginal zone lymphoma often affects the gastrointestinal tract. Its indolent nature combined with expected physiological ^{18}F-FDG uptake in organs such as the stomach may underscore ^{18}F-FDG PET/CT accuracy both at staging and upon treatment completion. Therefore, biopsies before and after treatment should be obtained to verify response to treatment [6].

Identification of bone marrow involvement is also crucial, especially in NHL, conferring an advanced stage disease status and often a poorer prognosis. Unilateral bone marrow biopsy (BMB) of the iliac crest evaluates a very limited part of the entire bone marrow compartment and false-negative cases may occur [27]. ¹⁸F-FDG PET/CT has demonstrated higher sensitivity in detecting bone marrow lymphomatous infiltration compared to BMB in both ¹⁸F-FDG-avid NHL and HD [28].

End-treatment ¹⁸F-FDG PET/CT in aggressive NHL and HD has proved to have high negative predictive value (NPV) differentiating viable tumor from residual fibrosis [29]. Nonetheless, false-positive results might occur, even when a window of 6–8 weeks after completion of chemotherapy and 8–12 weeks after radiotherapy has been respected. Therefore, serial ¹⁸F-FDG PET/CT scans may depict ¹⁸F-FDG uptake trend overtime or bioptic confirmation may be warranted in cases where further prompt treatment is recommended.

Finally, in cases where relapse is clinically suspected ¹⁸F-FDG PET/CT can support restaging and identification of an easily accessible lesion amenable to excisional biopsy if this hadn't yet been possible [30]. ¹⁸F-FDG PET/CT can guide a core biopsy or fine needle aspiration in deep-seated sites, avoiding necrotic or poorly cellulated parts of a bulky mass.

4.2 Histological Transformation

Indolent (low-grade) Non-Hodgkin lymphomas (NHL) include a variety of B and T cell lymphoproliferative disorders generally considered incurable. Indolent lymphomas progress slowly and treatment is focused on symptoms control when they become clinically significant: problems caused by enlarged lymph nodes, impending pancytopenia due to bone marrow infiltration, B-symptoms, etc [31, 32].

Follicular lymphoma grade I-II (FL I-II) is the most common and accounts for 70 % of all indolent lymphomas. Other frequent low-grade lymphomas are chronic lymphocytic leukemia or small lymphocytic lymphoma (CLL/SLL), lymphoplasmacytic lymphoma (LPL), nodal marginal zone lymphoma (MZL), splenic marginal zone lymphoma (SMZL), and mucosa-associated lymphoid tissue (MALT) lymphoma. Indolent lymphomas show variable, frequently poor, ¹⁸F-FDG uptake and guidelines from the National Comprehensive Cancer Network (NCCN) state that ¹⁸F-FDG PET/CT is useful in selected cases [1–3, 20, 31, 33, 34].

FL has a median survival of 8–10 years and, as other indolent lymphoproliferative disorders, can undergo histological transformation (HT) to a more aggressive type of lymphoma [32]. This is a well-known phenomenon that occurs in 5–10 % of patients and carries bad prognosis, with a short survival of less than 2 years [35, 36]. This situation has been extensively studied mostly in FL, which transforms to DLBCL and, less commonly, to BL or other types of aggressive lymphomas. Transformation can also be seen in other types of indolent lymphomas such as SLL/CLL transforming to either DLBCL (Richter's syndrome [RS]) or Hodgkin lymphoma. MALT or LPL and nodular-lymphocyte predominant HL (NLPHL) can transform to DLBCL and T-cell indolent lymphomas to high-grade T-cell lymphoma [32, 35].

HT is usually suspected in patients with low-grade lymphomas who develop rapidly growing adenopathies, B symptoms or LDH elevation. Identification of patients with HT requires a change in treatment strategy to intensified immuno-chemotherapy regimens that can eventually lead to a more favorable clinical response and better survival. Although it has not been extensively demonstrated that an earlier start of treatment can make a dramatic change in prognosis, there is consensus that it should be diagnosed and treated as soon as possible [32, 35].

Unfortunately, the pathogenesis of this biological transformation remains unclear, and it is not possible to predict which patients will develop this condition. Diagnosis of HT must rely on histological study, and ¹⁸F-FDG PET/CT can help identify lesions of higher metabolic activity than expected for indolent lymphomas that could be amenable for biopsy.

Schoder et al. [20] demonstrated in a study of 97 patients that an SUV >10 had sensitivity of 71 % and specificity of 81 % to predict an aggressive lymphoma and that an SUV >13 virtually excluded an indolent lymphoma. In 2009, in a study of 40 patients with transformed indolent lymphoma, Noy et al. found mean and median SUV max of biopsy proven transformed lesions of 14 and 12, respectively [25].

Bruzzi et al. [37] retrospectively studied 37 patients with CLL, 17 of which had clinical suspicion of HT. In this selected population, and using an SUV max cutoff value of 5, PET/CT demonstrated sensitivity, specificity, positive predictive value (PPV), and negative predictive value (NPV) of 91 %, 80 %, 53 %, and 97 % for Richter's transformation and 94 %, 90 %, 79 %, and 97 % for Richter's transformation, accelerated CLL, and/or detection of second malignancies.

Bodet-Milin et al. [38] analyzed 38 patients with indolent lymphoma and clinical suspicion of HT (FL, CLL, MZL, and Waldenström macroglobulinemia). They demonstrated a significant difference in SUV max in HT versus non-HT patients using histological confirmation of the site of highest ^{18}F-FDG uptake. Median SUV max was 18.5 (range, 11.7–41.2) in HT patients versus 8.6 (range, 1.7–17.0) in non-HT patients ($p < 0.0001$). The median SUV max was 13.7 (range, 6.1–37.3) in HT patients with HT versus 4.8 (range, 0.8–11.5) in non-HT patients ($p < 0.0001$). By ROC curve analysis, an SUV max of 14 showed a sensitivity and PPV of 93.9 % and a specificity and NPV of 95.3 % to differentiate HT from non-HT. An SUV max greater than 17 increased the PPV to 100 %, and an SUV max less than 11.7 increased the NPV to 100 %.

Tang et al. [34] studied 23 patients with FL and observed that there was a close correlation between metabolic activity and higher histopathological grade and Ki67, with a significant difference between grade I–II FL and grade III FL. Interestingly, in 61 % of patients, the site chosen for biopsy showed significant less metabolic activity measured in SUV than other lesions, suggesting existence of areas of transformation or higher proliferation index that might have been underestimated by sampling of a non-representative lesion.

Blase et al. [36] published a retrospective study on 88 patients with recently diagnosed indolent lymphomas (FL, CLL/SLL, LPL, MZL, MALT, hairy cell leukemia, and unspecified indolent lymphoma) staged with ^{18}F-FDG PET/CT. They found that in those patients whose lesions showed less or equal than normal liver parenchyma uptake, 100 % were free of HT up to 30 months of follow-up versus 88 % of patients whose lesions showed more uptake than normal liver parenchyma. In their population, LDH was also an independent predictor factor of transformation in uni- and multivariate analysis.

In summary, even though ^{18}F-FDG PET/CT is not commonly used in the evaluation of low-grade lymphoma patients, it might be useful in the setting of clinical suspicion of HT, specially to direct biopsy to the sites of highest ^{18}F-FDG uptake, allowing earlier diagnosis and treatment of HT.

4.3   Bone Marrow Involvement

Bone marrow infiltration/involvement (BMI) in lymphoma patients is diagnostic of stage IV disease requiring more aggressive treatment. BMI is diagnosed in 50–80 % of patients with low-grade NHL, 25–40 % of those with high-grade NHL and 5–14 % of those with HL. Its prevalence is less than 1 % among patients with early-stage high-grade disease, and bone marrow biopsy (BMB) is not routinely recommended in such patients in the absence of adverse prognostic factors [39].

Gold standard diagnostic procedure for BMI is uni- or bilateral iliac crest BMB, which is generally safe but can have complications (hemorrhage, infections) in about 0.12 % of cases. It is well known, however, that BMI is not necessarily generalized. In fact, it has been demonstrated in HL patients that bilateral iliac crest biopsy can increase procedure sensitivity by 10–22 %. For this reason it's generally accepted that a blind single sample in a specific site might miss neoplastic infiltration in other places [39–41].

^{18}F-FDG PET/CT imaging has gained an important role in the diagnosis of BMI in high grade lymphomas by allowing non-invasive visualization of the entire bone marrow and directing the biopsy to sites of high ^{18}F-FDG uptake [41].

El-Najjar et al. [40] published a review of the literature on the role of ^{18}F-FDG PET/CT and BMB in the staging of lymphoma patients. They concluded that ^{18}F-FDG PET/CT changes stage of patients in 18–45 % of cases (mostly because of upstaging) and modifies patient management in 11–38 % of the cases. However, it has a high rate of false negative studies for BMI in low grade lymphomas because of their frequent low metabolic activity and poor ^{18}F-FDG uptake that results in a sensitivity for detection of BMI in low grade lymphomas as low as 39 %. Therefore, they concluded that ^{18}F-FDG PET/CT is complementary to BMB, but cannot replace it.

In 2013, Adams et al published a meta-analysis that included nine studies with 955 patients with newly diagnosed HL who had all undergone staging with ^{18}F-FDG PET/CT. In this population, ^{18}F-FDG PET/CT showed a sensitivity and specificity for BMI of 96.9 % [95 % CI, 93.0–99.0 %] and 99.7 % (95 % CI, 98.9–100 %), respectively. The weighted summary proportion (fixed effects model) of ^{18}F-FDG PET/CT-negative patients with a positive BMB among all cases was 1.1 % (95 % CI, 0.6–2.0 %). They concluded that ^{18}F-FDG PET/CT could replace BMB in newly diagnosed HL patients [41].

In a retrospective study of 122 HL patients, Muzahir et al. [39] reported that ^{18}F-FDG PET/CT had sensitivity, specificity, NPV, PPV and accuracy of 100 %, 76.6 %, 76.6 %, 29.7 %, and 78.6 %, respectively, using bilateral iliac crest BMB as the reference standard. The authors also classified positive PET/CT studies into three different groups: diffuse BM uptake, unifocal BM uptake, or multifocal uptake. They found that only 18 % of patients with diffuse BM uptake had evidence of infiltration on biopsy and concluded that this uptake pattern is most probably secondary to cytokine-induced reactive bone marrow or inflammatory origin rather than neoplastic infiltration. However, the BMB was done consistently in the iliac crest in the 26 patients considered as to be false positives and not at the site of pathological ^{18}F-FDG uptake on the PET/CT study.

El-Galaly et al. [42] evaluated retrospectively 454 HL patients that were staged with ^{18}F-FDG PET/CT and unilateral iliac crest BMB from 2006 to 2011. Considering positive BMB and/or abnormal focal ^{18}F-FDG uptake that disappeared after chemotherapy consistent with BMI, they found sensitivity of 95 % (95 % CI, 86–99 %) for PET/CT versus 31 % (95 % CI, 22–42 %) for BMB and overall diagnostic accuracy of 99 % (95 % CI, 98–100 %) for PET/CT and 87 % (95 % CI, 84–90 %) for BMB. When considering only a positive BMB diagnostic for BMI, they found sensitivity, specificity, PPV, and NPV of focal skeletal PET/CT lesions for detection of BMI of 85 % (95 % CI, 66–96 %), 86 % (95 % CI, 83–89 %), 28 % (95 % CI, 19–39 %), and 99 % (95 % CI, 97–100 %), respectively. The authors concluded (1) that the added diagnostic value of routine BMB in HL patients who are undergoing ^{18}F-FDG PET/CT for staging was minimal, upstaging only 5 of 454 patients from stage III to stage IV, (2) that the low PPV of 28 % for prediction of BMI by ^{18}F-FDG PET/CT most probably reflected the large number of false-negative BMB results due to sampling errors rather than a high number of false-positive PET/CT results, and (3) that the high NPV of 99 % makes PET/CT a reliable tool for identifying patients in whom a BMB is not likely to add any diagnostic value.

Recently in January 2014, Cortes-Romera studied 147 high-grade lymphoma patients (84 with DLBCL, 63 with HL) staged with ^{18}F-FDG PET/CT and BMB and found sensitivity, specificity, accuracy, PPV, and NPV of ^{18}F-FDG PET/CT for the detection of BMI of 95 %, 86 %, 87 %, 54 %, and 99 %, respectively. ^{18}F-FDG PET/CT and BMB were concordant in 87 % of patients. Of 19 patients (13 %) were ^{18}F-FDG PET/CT and BMB were discordant, 18 had a positive ^{18}F-FDG PET/CT and a negative BMB biopsy not obtained in the hypermetabolic focus [43].

Adams et al. [44] published a systematic review and meta-analysis on ^{18}F-FDG PET/CT performance for diagnosis of BMI in DLBCL patients. They included seven studies published from 2008 to 2013 with a total of 654 patients and found a pooled sensitivity and specificity of

88.7 % (95 % CI, 82.5–93.3 %) and 99.8 % (95 % CI, 98.8–100 %), with an area under the ROC curve of 0.9983. The weighted summary proportion of ^{18}F-FDG PET/CT-negative patients with positive BMB was 3.1 % (95 % CI, 1.8–5.0 %) and of ^{18}F-FDG PET/CT-positive patients with negative BMB was 12.5 % (95 % CI, 8.4–17.3 %). The pooled sensitivity and specificity of ^{18}F-FDG PET/CT were 78.4 % (95 % CI, 69.9–85.5 %) and 99.7 % (95 % CI, 98.3–100 %) when focal bone marrow ^{18}F-FDG uptake was regarded as positive for BMI and 87.0 % (95 % CI, 79.2–92.7 %) and 100 % (95 % CI, 98.8–100 %) when both focal and diffuse bone marrow ^{18}F-FDG uptake were regarded as positive for BMI.

Finally, Berthet et al. studied 133 patients with newly diagnosed DLBCL who underwent ^{18}F-FDG PET/CT and unilateral iliac crest BMB for staging. ^{18}F-FDG PET/CT was considered positive when uni or multifocal abnormal bone marrow uptake was found, not explained by benign findings on CT. They found an accuracy of ^{18}F-FDG PET/CT for diagnosis of BMI of 97.7 % (95 % CI, 97.7–2.5 %), and for BMB of 81.2 % (95 % CI, 81.2–6.6 %). In this cohort they found just one false negative case for ^{18}F-FDG PET/CT (already stage IV for extranodal disease) and two false positives (one of which had a myeloproliferative disorder on BMB). They demonstrated a statistically significant higher sensitivity for ^{18}F-FDG PET/CT compared to BMB, 93.9 % versus 24.2 % ($P < 0.001$; 95 % CI, 93.9 % ± 8.1 % vs. 24.2 % ± 14.6 %), and NPV of 98 % for ^{18}F-FDG PET/CT versus 80 % for BMB (95 % CI, 98 % ± 2.7 % vs. 80 % ± 7 %). Both procedures showed similar specificity, 99 % versus 100 % (5 % CI, 99 % ± 1.9 % vs. 100 % ± 0 %) and PPV, 96.9 % versus 100 % (95 % CI, 96.9 % ± 6 % v/s 100 % ± 0 %) [28].

Current evidence shows that ^{18}F-FDG PET/CT is very accurate to diagnose BMI at initial staging of patients with high-grade lymphoma. It is a non-invasive procedure, allows visualization of the whole BM on axial and proximal appendicular skeleton and has very high sensitivity and NPV. False-positive cases using iliac crest BMB as the standard of reference probably reflects BMB sampling error

(biopsy not obtained in hypermetabolic focus), rather than real ^{18}F-FDG PET/CT false positives. Still, ^{18}F-FDG PET/CT can be falsely negative in approximately 3 % of cases. Therefore, in negative PET/CT studies, BMB should be performed if the bone marrow status will have prognostic and/or therapeutic implications. If ^{18}F-FDG PET/CT is positive for BMI, BMB may not be necessary.

In summary, ^{18}F-FDG PET/CT plays an important complementary role to BMB in the diagnosis of BMI in high-grade lymphomas (mostly HL and DLBCL). In indolent lymphomas, on the other hand, their frequent lower metabolic activity does not allow excluding BMI in ^{18}F-FDG PET/CT negative patients. At the time there is still no consensus on the ^{18}F-FDG uptake pattern that should be considered positive for BMI: diffuse, unifocal and/or multifocal pattern; or lower, equal or higher than normal liver uptake. A lot of research is still needed to draw some consensus on this issue.

Case 4.1

A 46-year-old male with a 4-month history of pruritus, night sweats, and fever.

^{18}F-FDG PET/CT findings: (a, b) Intense glycolytic activity is seen in several enlarged lymph nodes, above and below the diaphragm, and more prominent in the mediastinum and pulmonary hila. Several subcentimeter bilateral lung nodules have no significant ^{18}F-FDG uptake. (c) Hypermetabolic lung consolidation is noted at the left basis. Although suggestive of lymphomatous disease, a granulomatous process remains in the differential diagnosis and histological verification is necessary.

Biopsy: Mediastinal lymph node: Granulomatous inflammatory process, with fibrosing features, poorly necrotizing consistent with sarcoidosis. No cultural growth of fungi, bacteria, or mycobacteria. Polymerase chain reaction was negative for mycobacteria.

Recommendations: ^{18}F-FDG PET/CT cannot be used to formulate the initial diagnosis of lymphoma since non-oncological processes and other malignancies can mimic lymphoma appearances on ^{18}F-FDG PET imaging.

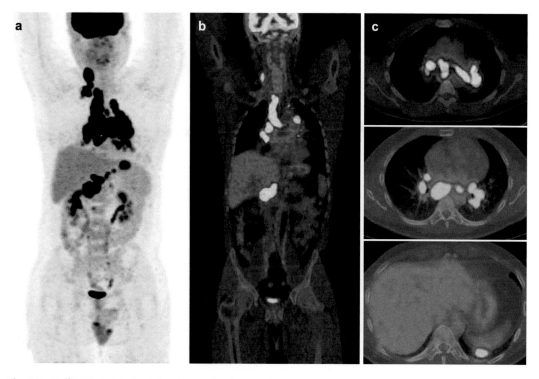

Fig. 4.1 (**a**) ¹⁸F-FDG MIP, (**b**, **c**) fused coronal and transaxial images of the thorax

Case 4.2

A 60-year-old male with enlarged cervical, axillary, and inguinal lymphadenopathy.

¹⁸F-FDG PET/CT findings: (a, b) Moderately ¹⁸F-FDG-avid lymphadenopathy is noted in the bilateral cervical, supraclavicular, and axillary basins, as well as mild splenomegaly with ¹⁸F-FDG activity slightly above liver uptake. (a, b, c) Mediastinal lymph nodes as well as retroperitoneal, iliac, and inguinal regions bilaterally show mild ¹⁸F-FDG uptake.

Biopsy:

- Excisional left cervical node biopsy reveals small lymphocytic lymphoma with features of high-grade lymphoma transformation.
- Bone marrow biopsy: Infiltration by small lymphocytic lymphoma. Stage IV.

Recommendation: Staging of a low-grade lymphoma with suspicious transformation to a more aggressive histological type. ¹⁸F-FDG PET/CT can guide biopsy to high-grade lymphadenopathy. ¹⁸F-FDG PET/CT could not detect bone marrow infiltration by the low-grade lymphoma.

Case 4.3

A 60-year-old patient recently diagnosed with anaplastic T-cell non-Hodgkin lymphoma.

¹⁸F-FDG PET/CT findings: (a, b) Solid mass with homogeneous high ¹⁸F-FDG uptake in the left-sided anterior mediastinum extending to the left pulmonary hilum. Small ¹⁸F-FDG-avid nodes are noted above and below the diaphragm. Intense ¹⁸F-FDG activity is noted at the left apical pleura. (c) Moderately hypermetabolic foci can be seen at multiple bone marrow sites. Conclusion: supradiaphragmatic nodal disease and patchy bone marrow infiltration (stage IV).

Biopsy: Right laterocervical lymph node, anaplastic T-cell non-Hodgkin lymphoma.

Bone marrow biopsy from the left iliac crest showed no disease.

Recommendations: ¹⁸F-FDG PET/CT is the gold standard for staging high-grade NHL. In this case, bone marrow biopsy performed on the iliac

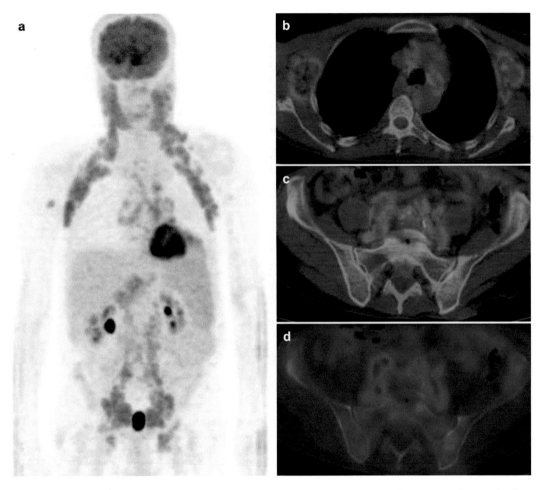

Fig. 4.2 (**a**) ^{18}F-FDG MIP; fused transaxial images of (**b**) axillary basins; (**c**) common iliac basins; (**d**) posterior iliac crests

crest showed no involvement; however, scattered focal areas of increased ^{18}F-FDG uptake can be seen in other bone marrow segments highly suspicious for bone marrow involvement.

Case 4.4

A 31-year-old male with newly diagnosed diffuse large B-cell lymphoma.

^{18}F-FDG PET/CT findings: (a, b, c) Mediastinal bulky mass with heterogeneous ^{18}F-FDG uptake, mainly peripheral, as well as small hypermetabolic lymph nodes in the right subclavian and left para-aortic regions. (d) Extranodal intense ^{18}F-FDG-avid lesions in both adrenals, head of the pancreas, the greater gastric

curvature, and the right kidney. Conclusion: stage IV partly necrotic mediastinal bulky mass with extranodal involvement (adrenals, head of the pancreas, right kidney, stomach).

Biopsy: Diffuse large B-cell lymphoma

Recommendations: Staging aggressive NHL. ^{18}F-FDG PET/CT scan can guide biopsy to site of high ^{18}F-FDG uptake in a bulky mass. At staging ^{18}F-FDG PET/CT contributes to prognostication in terms of Ann Arbor status and extranodal involvement (IPI score).

Case 4.5

A 62-year-old male with marginal zone lymphoma.

^{18}F-FDG PET/CT findings: (a) Mild focal increased ^{18}F-FDG uptake in the left upper quadrant;

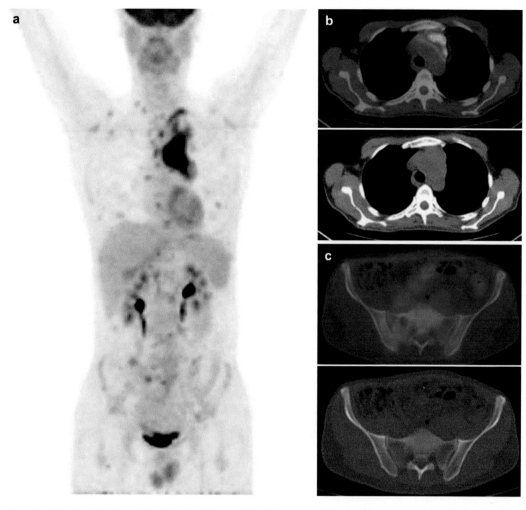

Fig. 4.3 (**a**) ¹⁸F-FDG MIP; (**b**) fused ¹⁸F-FDG PET/CT and low-dose CT transaxial images of the mediastinum; (**c**) fused ¹⁸F-FDG PET/CT and low-dose CT transaxial images of the pelvis

(b) ¹⁸F-FDG PET, CT, and fusion transaxial images of the abdomen show a small focus of mildly increased ¹⁸F-FDG uptake in the gastric fundus, suggestive of low-grade lymphoma.

Biopsy: Endoscopic gastric biopsy: MALT lymphoma (extranodal marginal zone lymphoma of mucosa-associated lymphoid tissues).

Recommendations: Low-grade lymphomas frequently show variable, most frequently poor, ¹⁸F-FDG uptake.

Case 4.6

A 62-year-old female with grade I follicular lymphoma on observation since 2012. She presents with a 2-month history of fever and LDH elevation.

¹⁸F-FDG PET/CT findings: (a, b, c) Multiple bilateral small nodes with low ¹⁸F-FDG uptake in the neck, supraclavicular and axillary regions, right internal mammary chain and mediastinum, and mildly hypometabolic dorsal subcutaneous nodule, SUV max 3.5. (d, e) Intensely ¹⁸F-FDG-avid adenopathy in the left external iliac and inguinal regions, SUV max 11.2 (thin arrow), and small hypometabolic lymph nodes in the right iliac and inguinal chains (arrow head), similar to those seen in the neck and thorax.

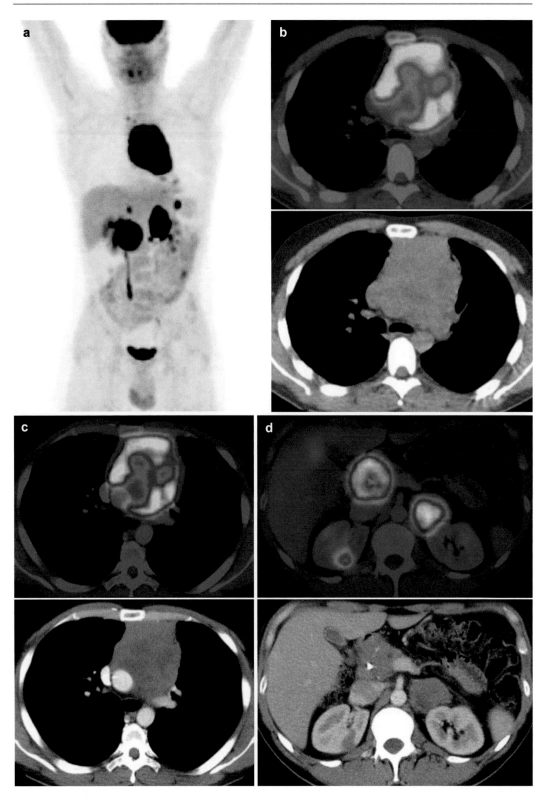

Fig. 4.4 (**a**) ¹⁸F-FDG MIP; (**b**) fused ¹⁸F-FDG PET/CT and low-dose CT transaxial images of the mediastinum; (**c**) fused ¹⁸F-FDG PET/CECT and CECT transaxial images of the mediastinum (**d**) fused PET/CECT and CECT transaxial images of the upper abdomen

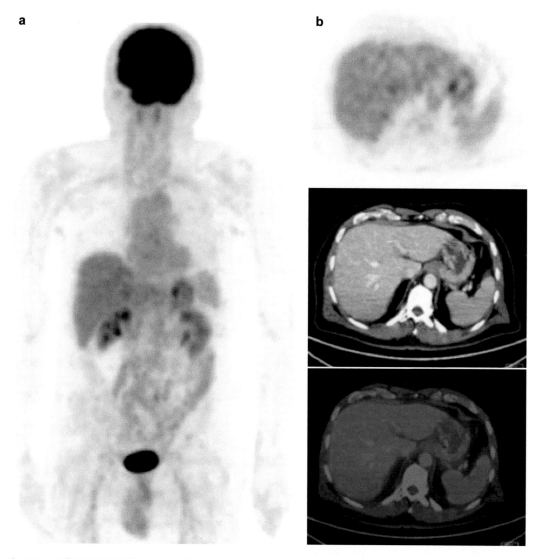

Fig. 4.5 (**a**) ^{18}F-FDG PET/CT MIP; (**b**) ^{18}F-FDG PET, CECT, and fusion transaxial images of the abdomen

Biopsy: Excisional biopsy of the left inguinal adenopathy with high ^{18}F-FDG uptake demonstrated high-grade lymphoproliferative disorder, compatible with follicular lymphoma G3, most probably arising from an underlying low-grade follicular lymphoma (histological transformation).

Recommendation: Given that patient prognosis and therapeutic regimens are determined by the most aggressive disease, histological study should be obtained in the lesion with the highest ^{18}F-FDG uptake.

Case 4.7
A 63-year-old female with marginal zone lymphoma.

^{18}F-FDG PET/CT findings November 2010: (a, b) Small right axillary lymph nodes with low-grade ^{18}F-FDG uptake, SUV max 2.3, consistent with the diagnosis of marginal zone lymphoma (low grade).

^{18}F-FDG PET/CT findings May 2012: (c) Multiple supra- and infradiaphragmatic foci of intense pathological hypermetabolism; (d, e) cervical and retroperitoneal lymph nodes with intense ^{18}F-FDG uptake, SUV max 24.5; (f, g)

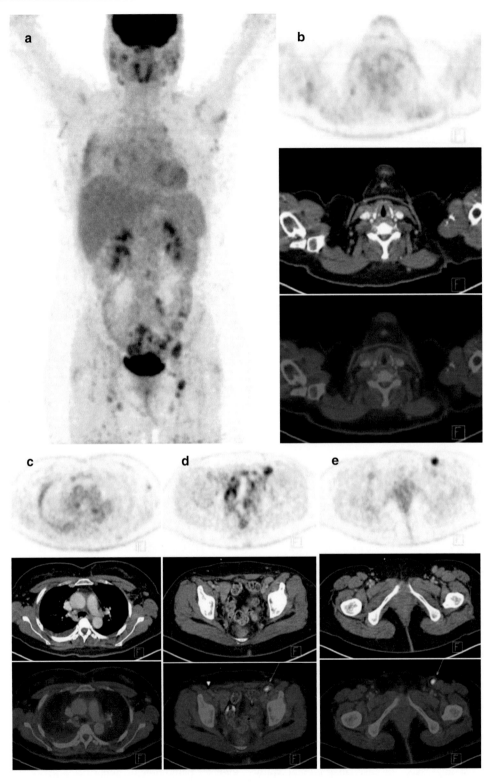

Fig. 4.6 (a) ^{18}F-FDG PET/CT MIP; (b–e) ^{18}F-FDG PET, CECT, and fused transaxial images of the neck, thorax, pelvis, and inguinal regions

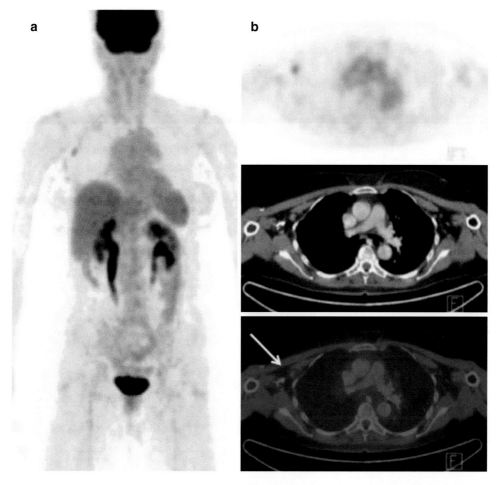

Fig. 4.7 (a) ^{18}F-FDG PET/CT MIP; (b) ^{18}F-FDG PET, CECT, and fused transaxial images of the thorax, November 2010

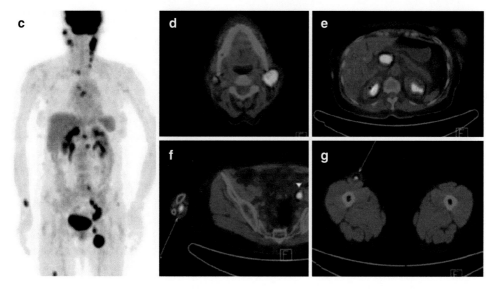

Fig. 4.7 (c) ^{18}F-FDG PET/CT MIP; (d–g) ^{18}F-FDG PET/CT-fused transaxial images of the neck, abdomen, pelvis, and thighs, May 2012

abnormal ¹⁸F-FDG uptake in external iliac lymph node (arrow head) and in soft tissue nodules intramuscular in the right arm and subcutaneous in the right thigh (thin arrows), SUV max 7.8.

Appearance of multiple supra- and infradiaphragmatic hypermetabolic lesions is highly suspicious for histological transformation of low-grade lymphoma.

Biopsy: Excisional biopsy of the left cervical adenopathy with high ¹⁸F-FDG uptake demonstrated transformed high-grade large B-cell lymphoma.

Recommendation: Low-grade lymphoma patients, who develop high metabolic activity lesions, should undergo histological study to evaluate possible histological transformation to aggressive lymphoma or a different neoplastic/non-neoplastic origin.

Case 4.8

A 57-year-old male with newly diagnosed DLBCL.

¹⁸F-FDG PET/CT findings: (a) ¹⁸F-FDG PET/CT MIP shows multiple pathological supra- and infradiaphragmatic foci of abnormal ¹⁸F-FDG uptake; (b, c, d and e) intense pathological ¹⁸F-FDG uptake in the left lung nodule, liver lesions, right kidney cortex, and left femoral neck bone marrow, with no abnormal findings on CT in this last location.

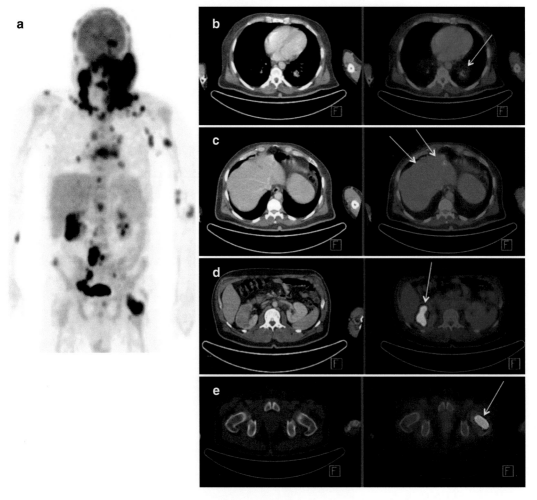

Fig. 4.8 (**a**) ¹⁸F-FDG PET/CT MIP; (**b–e**) ¹⁸F-FDG PET, CECT, and fusion transaxial images of the thorax, abdomen, and pelvis

Biopsy: Excisional biopsy of cervical adenopathy showed a diffuse large B-cell lymphoma. Interestingly, BMB of the iliac crest was negative in this patient.

Interpretation: Intense pathological ¹⁸F-FDG uptake in lymph nodes, solid organs, soft tissues, and skeleton compatible with extensive stage IV disease. Abnormal bone marrow ¹⁸F-FDG uptake with no abnormal findings on CT is highly suggestive of bone marrow infiltration by high-grade lymphoma, regardless of a negative iliac crest bone marrow biopsy (most probably a false-negative bone marrow biopsy due to sampling error).

References

1. Swerdlow SH, Campo E, Harris NL, Jaffe ES, Pileri SA, Stein H, Thiele J, editors. WHO classification of tumours of haematopoietic and lymphoid tissues. Lyon: IARC; 2008.
2. NCCN Clinical Practice Guidelines in Oncology: Hodgkin Lymphoma Version 2. 2013. http://www.nccn.org.
3. NCCN Clinical Practice Guidelines in Oncology: Non-Hodgkin Lymphoma Version 2. 2013. http://www.nccn.org.
4. Engert A, Eichenauer DA, Dreyling M, ESMO Guidelines Working Group. Hodgkin's lymphoma: ESMO Clinical Practice Guidelines for diagnosis, treatment and follow-up. Ann Oncol. 2010;21 Suppl 5:v168–71.
5. Dreyling M, Ghielmini M, Marcus R, Salles G, Vitolo U. Newly diagnosed and relapsed follicular lymphoma: ESMO Clinical Practice Guidelines for diagnosis, treatment and follow-up. Ann Oncol. 2011;22 Suppl 6:vi59–63.
6. Zucca E, Dreyling M, ESMO Guidelines Working Group. Gastric marginal zone lymphoma of MALT type: ESMO Clinical Practice Guidelines for diagnosis, treatment and follow-up. Ann Oncol. 2010;21 Suppl 5:v175–6.
7. Tilly H, Dreyling M, ESMO Guidelines Working Group. Diffuse large B-cell non-Hodgkin's lymphoma: ESMO Clinical Practice Guidelines for diagnosis, treatment and follow-up. Ann Oncol. 2010;21 Suppl 5:v172–4.
8. Li JY, Gaillard F, Moreau A, Harousseau JL, Laboisse C, Milpied N, Bataille R, Avet-Loiseau H. Detection of translocation t(11;14)(q13;q32) in mantle cell lymphoma by fluorescence in situ hybridization. Am J Pathol. 1999;154(5):1449–52.
9. Horn H, Ziepert M, Becher C, Barth TF, Bernd HW, Feller AC, Klapper W, Hummel M, Stein H, Hansmann ML, Schmelter C, Möller P, Cogliatti S,

Pfreundschuh M, Schmitz N, Trümper L, Siebert R, Loeffler M, Rosenwald A, Ott G, German High-Grade Non-Hodgkin Lymphoma Study Group. MYC status in concert with BCL2 and BCL6 expression predicts outcome in diffuse large B-cell lymphoma. Blood. 2013;121(12):2253–63.
10. Sehn LH. Paramount prognostic factors that guide therapeutic strategies in diffuse large B-cell lymphoma. Hematol Am Soc Hematol Educ Program. 2012;2012:402–9.
11. Alizadeh AA, Eisen MB, Davis RE, Ma C, Lossos IS, Rosenwald A, Boldrick JC, Sabet H, Tran T, Yu X, Powell JI, Yang L, Marti GE, Moore T, Hudson Jr J, Lu L, Lewis DB, Tibshirani R, Sherlock G, Chan WC, Greiner TC, Weisenburger DD, Armitage JO, Warnke R, Levy R, Wilson W, Grever MR, Byrd JC, Botstein D, Brown PO, Staudt LM. Distinct types of diffuse large B-cell lymphoma identified by gene expression profiling. Nature. 2000;403(6769):503–11.
12. Liu H, Ruskon-Fourmestraux A, Lavergne-Slove A, Ye H, Molina T, Bouhnik Y, Hamoudi RA, Diss TC, Dogan A, Megraud F, Rambaud JC, Du MQ, Isaacson PG. Resistance of t(11;18) positive gastric mucosa-associated lymphoid tissue lymphoma to Helicobacter pylori eradication therapy. Lancet. 2001;357(9249): 39–40.
13. Barrena S, Almeida J, Del Carmen García-Macias M, López A, Rasillo A, Sayagués JM, Rivas RA, Gutiérrez ML, Ciudad J, Flores T, Balanzategui A, Caballero MD, Orfao A. Flow cytometry immunophenotyping of fine-needle aspiration specimens: utility in the diagnosis and classification of non-Hodgkin lymphomas. Histopathology. 2011;58(6):906–18.
14. Paes FM, Kalkanis DG, Sideras PA, Serafini AN. FDG PET/CT of extranodal involvement in non-Hodgkin lymphoma and Hodgkin disease. Radiographics. 2010;30(1):269–91.
15. Kostakoglu L, Cheson BD. State-of-the-art research on "lymphomas: role of molecular imaging for staging, prognostic evaluation, and treatment response". Front Oncol. 2013;3:212. eCollection 2013. Review.
16. Cheson BD. Role of functional imaging in the management of lymphoma. J Clin Oncol. 2011;29(14): 1844–54. doi:10.1200/JCO.2010.32.5225. Epub 2011 Apr 11. Review. Erratum in: J Clin Oncol. 2011; 29(19):2739.
17. Le Dortz L, De Guibert S, Bayat S, Devillers A, Houot R, Rolland Y, Cuggia M, Le Jeune F, Bahri H, Barge ML, Lamy T, Garin E. Diagnostic and prognostic impact of 18F-FDG PET/CT in follicular lymphoma. Eur J Nucl Med Mol Imaging. 2010; 37(12):2307–14.
18. Hutchings M. How does PET/CT help in selecting therapy for patients with Hodgkin lymphoma? Hematol Am Soc Hematol Educ Program. 2012; 2012:322–7. doi:10.1182/asheducation-2012.1.322. Review. PubMed.
19. Kako S, Izutsu K, Ota Y, Minatani Y, Sugaya M, Momose T, et al. FDG-PET in T-cell and NK-cell neoplasms. Ann Oncol Off J Eur Soc Med Oncol ESMO. 2007;18(10):1685–90.

20. Schöder H, Noy A, Gönen M, Weng L, Green D, Erdi YE, Larson SM, Yeung HW. Intensity of 18fluorode-oxyglucose uptake in positron emission tomography distinguishes between indolent and aggressive non-Hodgkin's lymphoma. J Clin Oncol. 2005;23(21):4643–51.

21. Weiler-Sagie M, Bushelev O, Epelbaum R, Dann EJ, Haim N, Avivi I, Ben-Barak A, Ben-Arie Y, Bar-Shalom R, Israel O. (18)F-FDG avidity in lymphoma readdressed: a study of 766 patients. J Nucl Med. 2010;51(1):25–30.

22. Wirth A, Foo M, Seymour JF, Macmanus MP, Hicks RJ. Impact of [18f] fluorodeoxyglucose positron emission tomography on staging and management of early-stage follicular non-hodgkin lymphoma. Int J Radiat Oncol Biol Phys. 2008;71(1):213–9.

23. Luminari S, Biasoli I, Arcaini L, Versari A, Rusconi C, Merli F, Spina M, Ferreri AJ, Zinzani PL, Gallamini A, Mastronardi S, Boccomini C, Gaidano G, D'Arco AM, Di Raimondo F, Carella AM, Santoro A, Musto P, Federico M. The use of FDG-PET in the initial staging of 142 patients with follicular lymphoma: a retrospective study from the FOLL05 randomized trial of the Fondazione Italiana Linfomi. Ann Oncol. 2013;24(8):2108–12.

24. Bodet-Milin C, Touzeau C, Leux C, Sahin M, Moreau A, Maisonneuve H, Morineau N, Jardel H, Moreau P, Gallazini-Crépin C, Gries P, Gressin R, Harousseau JL, Mohty M, Moreau P, Kraeber-Bodere F, Le Gouill S. Prognostic impact of 18F-fluoro-deoxyglucose positron emission tomography in untreated mantle cell lymphoma: a retrospective study from the GOELAMS group. Eur J Nucl Med Mol Imaging. 2010;37(9):1633–42.

25. Noy A, Schöder H, Gönen M, Weissler M, Ertelt K, Cohler C, Portlock C, Hamlin P, Yeung HW. The majority of transformed lymphomas have high standardized uptake values (SUVs) on positron emission tomography (PET) scanning similar to diffuse large B-cell lymphoma (DLBCL). Ann Oncol. 2009;20(3):508–12.

26. Castellucci P, Nanni C, Farsad M, Alinari L, Zinzani P, Stefoni V, Battista G, Valentini D, Pettinato C, Marengo M, Boschi S, Canini R, Baccarani M, Monetti N, Franchi R, Rampin L, Fanti S, Rubello D. Potential pitfalls of 18F-FDG PET in a large series of patients treated for malignant lymphoma: prevalence and scan interpretation. Nucl Med Commun. 2005;26(8):689–94.

27. Schaefer NG, Strobel K, Taverna C, Hany TF. Bone involvement in patients with lymphoma: the role of FDG-PET/CT. Eur J Nucl Med Mol Imaging. 2007;34(1):60–7.

28. Berthet L, Cochet A, Kanoun S, Berriolo-Riedinger A, Humbert O, Toubeau M, Dygai-Cochet I, Legouge C, Casasnovas O, Brunotte F. In newly diagnosed diffuse large B-cell lymphoma, determination of bone marrow involvement with 18F-FDG PET/CT provides better diagnostic performance and prognostic stratification than does biopsy. J Nucl Med. 2013;54(8):1244–50.

29. Terasawa T, Nihashi T, Hotta T, Nagai H. 18F-FDG PET for posttherapy assessment of Hodgkin's disease and aggressive Non-Hodgkin's lymphoma: a systematic review. J Nucl Med. 2008;49(1):13–21.

30. Cerci JJ, Pereira Neto CC, Krauzer C, Sakamoto DG, Vitola JV. The impact of coaxial core biopsy guided by FDG PET/CT in oncological patients. Eur J Nucl Med Mol Imaging. 2013;40(1):98–103.

31. Cronin CG, Swords R, Truong MT, Viswanathan C, Rohren E, Giles FJ, O'Dwyer M, Bruzzi JF. Clinical utility of PET/CT in lymphoma. AJR Am J Roentgenol. 2010;194(1):W91–103.

32. Montoto S, Fitzgibbon J. Transformation of indolent B-cell lymphomas. J Clin Oncol. 2011;29(14):1827–34.

33. Okada M, Sato N, Ishii K, Matsumura K, Hosono M, Murakami T. FDG PET/CT versus CT, MR imaging, and 67Ga scintigraphy in the posttherapy evaluation of malignant lymphoma. Radiographics. 2010;30(4):939–57.

34. Tang B, Malysz J, Douglas-Nikitin V, Zekman R, Wong RH, Jaiyesimi I, Wong CY. Correlating metabolic activity with cellular proliferation in follicular lymphomas. Mol Imaging Biol. 2009;11(5):296–302.

35. Al-Tourah AJ, Gill KK, Chhanabhai M, Hoskins PJ, Klasa RJ, Savage KJ, Sehn LH, Shenkier TN, Gascoyne RD, Connors JM. Population-based analysis of incidence and outcome of transformed non-Hodgkin's lymphoma. J Clin Oncol. 2008;26(32):5165–9.

36. Blase PE, Pasker-de Jong PCM, Hagenbeek A, Fijnheer R, de Haas M, de Klerk JMH. Predictive potential of FDG-PET/CT for histological transformation in patients with indolent lymphoma. Adv Mol Imaging. 2014;4:1–10.

37. Bruzzi JF, Macapinlac H, Tsimberidou AM, Truong MT, Keating MJ, Marom EM, Munden RF. Detection of Richter's transformation of chronic lymphocytic leukemia by PET/CT. J Nucl Med. 2006;47(8):1267–73.

38. Bodet-Milin C, Kraeber-Bodéré F, Moreau P, Campion L, Dupas B, Le Gouill S. Investigation of FDG-PET/CT imaging to guide biopsies in the detection of histological transformation of indolent lymphoma. Haematologica. 2008;93(3):471–2.

39. Muzahir S, Mian M, Munir I, Nawaz MK, Faruqui ZS, Mufti KA, Bashir H, Uddin N, Siddiqui N, Maaz AU, Mahmood MT. Clinical utility of 18F FDG-PET/CT in the detection of bone marrow disease in Hodgkin's lymphoma. Br J Radiol. 2012;85(1016):e490–6.

40. El-Najjar I, Barwick T, Avril N, Montoto S. The role of FDG-PET and bone marrow examination in lymphoma staging. Ann Oncol. 2012;23 Suppl 10:x89–91. PubMed.

41. Adams HJ, Kwee TC, de Keizer B, Fijnheer R, de Klerk JM, Littooij AS, Nievelstein RA. Systematic review and meta-analysis on the diagnostic

performance of FDG-PET/CT in detecting bone marrow involvement in newly diagnosed Hodgkin lymphoma: is bone marrow biopsy still necessary? Ann Oncol. 2014;25(5):921–7.

42. El-Galaly TC, d'Amore F, Mylam KJ, de Brown Nully P, Bøgsted M, Bukh A, Specht L, Loft A, Iyer V, Hjorthaug K, Nielsen AL, Christiansen I, Madsen C, Johnsen HE, Hutchings M. Routine bone marrow biopsy has little or no therapeutic consequence for positron emission tomography/computed tomography-staged treatment-naive patients with Hodgkin lymphoma. J Clin Oncol. 2012;30(36):4508–14.

43. Cortés-Romera M, Sabaté-Llobera A, Mercadal-Vilchez S, Climent-Esteller F, Serrano-Maestro A, Gámez-Cenzano C, González-Barca E. Bone marrow evaluation in initial staging of lymphoma: 18F-FDG PET/CT versus bone marrow biopsy. Clin Nucl Med. 2014;39(1):e46–52.

44. Adams HJ, Kwee TC, de Keizer B, Fijnheer R, de Klerk JM, Nievelstein RA. FDG PET/CT for the detection of bone marrow involvement in diffuse large B-cell lymphoma: systematic review and meta-analysis. Eur J Nucl Med Mol Imaging. 2014; 41(3):565–74.

Francesco Ceci, Paolo Castelluci,
and Tiziano Graziani

5.1 Introduction

Prostate cancer (PC) is the most common cancer in men and the third leading cause of death in economically developed countries. Its incidence rate in the European Union has increased to 78.9 per 100,000 per year with a mortality rate of 30.6 per 100,000 per year [1]. Prostate cancer can be a clinically silent and/or indolent intra-prostatic disease or very aggressive.

Suspicion for prostate cancer is most commonly based on digital rectal examination (DRE), serum levels of prostate-specific antigen (PSA) and transrectal ultrasound (TRUS) [2].

The standard of reference is histopathological examination of prostate tissue, which can be obtained by fine-needle prostate TRUS-guided biopsy [3]. When histology confirms the presence of prostate cancer, patients can be staged with imaging procedures to evaluate tumour extension and to assess the presence of a distant spread [4].

Transrectal ultrasound (TRUS), magnetic resonance (MR), computerized tomography (CT) and bone scintigraphy (BS) are established imaging modalities to study PC patients. Functional imaging with positron emission tomography (PET) provides additional information compared to conventional imaging (CI) [5]. Several PET radiopharmaceuticals have been investigated for PC imaging such as ^{18}F-FDG, ^{11}C-acetate [6] and ^{18}F-fluoroacetate, ^{18}F-fluorodihydrotestosterone (FDHT) [7], ^{11}C-methionine [8] and ^{68}Ga-DOTANOC [9].

Choline labelled with ^{11}C or ^{18}F is the most promising for the diagnosis, staging and restaging of prostate cancer patients. Choline is a substrate for phosphatidylcholine synthesis, which is the major phospholipid in the cell membrane. The use of choline for PET/CT imaging of PC is based on up-regulation of the choline metabolism in tumour cells due to increased activity of the enzyme choline kinase [10]. In addition, choline uptake is related to a membrane-selective transporter [11], which is increased in prostate cancer cells too. Choline can be labelled with ^{11}C or ^{18}F: the main difference between the two tracers is the earlier urinary appearance of the ^{18}F-choline, probably due to incomplete tubular reuptake [12]. This is particularly relevant in prostate cancer diagnosis, staging and assessment of local relapse since sensitivity of the procedure in the pelvis can be reduced by the presence of radioactive urine in the bladder. On the other hand, ^{11}C has a half-life of 20 min and it has to be used soon after production. This is the main limitation of ^{11}C agents, requiring

F. Ceci, MD (✉) • P. Castelluci, MD
T. Graziani, MD
Service of Nuclear Medicine, Dipartimento di
Medicina Specialistica, Diagnostica e Sperimentale,
Azienda Ospedaliero-Universitaria
Policlinico S.Orsola-Malpighi,
University of Bologna, Bologna, Italy
e-mail: francesco.ceci83@gmail.com

© Springer International Publishing 2016
J. Cerci et al. (eds.), *Oncological PET/CT with Histological Confirmation*,
DOI 10.1007/978-3-319-27880-3_5

the presence of an on-site cyclotron. ^{18}F-labelled choline tracers, with a 110 min half-life, are under development.

5.2   Choline PET/CT to Guide Biopsy for Prostate Cancer

The initial approach to prostate cancer diagnosis is mostly based on DRE and/or serum levels of PSA, followed by TRUS-guided biopsy [13–16]. However, these imaging modalities show some limitations. TRUS-guided biopsy is false negative and/or non-diagnostic in up to 30–40 % of patients with prostate cancer. In patients with large prostates or with unusual location of cancer, TRUS-guided biopsy is commonly performed more than twice before demonstrating malignant cells. This leads to 3–4 months delay in diagnosis and a higher risk of co-morbidity [17–19]. As the main limitations of serum levels of PSA are the lack of specificity and precise localization, other imaging modalities have been investigated and it showed that CT has limited accuracy in the diagnosis of the primary tumour, because differentiation between normal, benign prostatic tissue and malignancy is not always possible. MR with endo-rectal coil and spectroscopy has the highest accuracy among the CI modalities in the evaluation of intra-prostatic cancer [20–22], in particular in association with three-dimensional (3D) MR spectroscopic imaging [13]. Limitations of this technique are low accuracy if performed after biopsy and limited availability in many diagnostic centres [23, 24].

Therefore, the potential role of choline PET/CT in the diagnosis of PC has been investigated, in order to establish if it could increase the TRUS-guided biopsy sensitivity in patients with high risk of disease and multiple non-diagnostic biopsies and/or guide the biopsy. Several studies demonstrate controversial results, as reviewed recently by Farsad et al. [25]. The first study was performed by De Jong et al. [26]. The authors assessed the detection of primary tumour with ^{11}C-choline PET in patients with biopsy-proven prostate cancer compared with patients with benign prostatic disease. In the benign prostatic tissue, the SUVmean was 2.3 (1.3–3.2), while it was 5.0 (2.4–9.5) in malignant tissue. There was focal ^{11}C-choline uptake in 24 of 25 patients with prostate cancer.

The first study on sextant-based comparison with histology was performed by Farsad et al. [27], who investigated the potential usefulness of ^{11}C-choline PET/CT for detection and localization of tumours within the prostate in 36 patients before surgery. Histopathology analysis detected prostate cancer in 143/216 sextants, high-grade prostate intraepithelial neoplasm (HGPIN) in 89/216 sextants (59/89 sextants associated with cancer cells, 30/89 sextants not associated with cancer cells) and acute prostatitis in 7/216 sextants (3/4 sextants with associated cancer cells, 1/4 sextants not associated with cancer cells), and 39/216 sextants were normal. ^{11}C-choline PET/CT showed a sensitivity of 66 %, a specificity of 81 %, an accuracy of 71 %, a positive predictive value (PPV) of 87 % and a negative predictive value (NPV) of 55 %. In conclusion, ^{11}C-choline PET/CT was able to demonstrate foci of prostate cancer but with a high rate of false negative on a sextant basis.

Reske et al. [28] studied 26 PC patients with ^{11}C-choline PET/CT and reported that regions with PC were identified in all patients, with a sensitivity of 100 % and specificity of 87 %. The authors found that a SUVmax cut-off of 2.65 resulted in AUC of 0.89 ± 0.01 in the ROC analysis for a correct prediction of the disease. The authors reported a significant higher ^{11}C-choline uptake in prostate cancer compared to normal prostatic tissue, prostatitis or HGPIN ($p < 0.001$). No correlations were found between ^{11}C-choline PET/CT SUV and PSA value, Gleason score, but a correlation with T stage was observed.

Giovacchini et al. [29] performed a study on 19 patients in which they compared ^{11}C-choline PET/CT with post-prostatectomy histopathologic axial step sections. They found a sensitivity of 72 % and specificity of 43 % using a SUVmax cut-off of 2.5 to differentiate benign and malignant lesions. The authors found that coexistence of prostatitis, HGPIN and benign prostatic hyperplasia (BPH) was a main limitation of their study.

Martorana et al. [30] performed a comparison between the sensitivity of ^{11}C-choline PET/CT and 12-core transrectal biopsy in 43 patients with established prostate cancer before initial biopsy. ^{11}C-choline PET/CT showed a sensitivity of 83 % in the detection on nodule ≥5 mm, but 4 % for lesions <5 mm. The tumour size was the only factor that influenced ^{11}C-choline PET/CT detection. At sextant analysis, ^{11}C-choline PET/CT showed a slightly better sensitivity than TRUS (66 % vs 61 %) but less specificity (84 % vs 97 %).

Several studies in literature compared MR and ^{11}C-choline PET/CT. One of these was performed by Testa et al. [31]. They retrospectively compared the sensitivity and specificity of MR, (3D) MR spectroscopy, MR associated with and 3D MR spectroscopy and ^{11}C-choline PET/CT for intra-prostatic tumour sextant localization, with histologic findings as reference standard. The sensitivity, specificity and accuracy were, respectively, 55 %, 86 % and 67 % with ^{11}C-choline PET/CT; 54 %, 75 % and 61 % with MR imaging; and 81 %, 67 % and 76 % with 3D MR spectroscopy. The highest sensitivity was obtained when either 3D MR spectroscopic or MR imaging results were positive (88 %) at the expense of specificity (53 %), while the highest specificity was obtained when results with both techniques were positive (90 %) at the expense of sensitivity (48 %). Concordance between 3D MR spectroscopic and ^{11}C-choline PET/CT findings was limited.

In conclusion, choline PET/CT cannot be recommended as first-line screening imaging procedure in patients with high risk of prostate cancer. Choline PET/CT has moderate sensitivity, which is related to the tumour configuration. The sensitivity of choline PET/CT is negatively influenced by the presence of microcarcinoma below the limits of PET resolution. The specificity of choline PET/CT is limited as the spectrum of differentiation between benign prostatic changes (prostatitis, HGPIN, BPH) and malignant tissue.

However, considering the limitations of the other imaging procedures (TRUS, MR, CT) for the diagnosis of PC, choline PET/CT has a role to guide TRUS biopsy, the site of higher uptake visualized by the choline PET/CT in patients with clinically suspected prostate cancer and at least two consecutive negative prostate biopsies.

5.3   Clinical Cases

Case 5.1

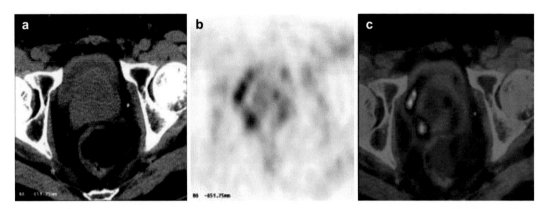

This 65-year-old man (R.S.) had a TRUS-guided biopsy on October 2007 for suspicion of prostate cancer based on a high serum PSA level of 12 ng/mL and an increased total volume of the prostate gland described at TRUS and DRE. The biopsy was negative/non-diagnostic for malignant cells. After 3 months, the PSA raised up to 21 ng/mL, and the patient was referred for another biopsy that was again negative/non-diagnostic. On March 2008, a ^{11}C-choline PET/CT was performed (A low-dose CT, B PET, C fusion images). A focus of higher uptake of choline was observed at the right base of the prostate. Low-dose CT confirmed increased dimension of the prostate gland. A third TRUS-guided biopsy was performed, guided to the focus of ^{11}C-choline uptake. The histological examination confirmed the presence of a prostate cancer cells with a Gleason score of 4 + 3.

Case 5.2

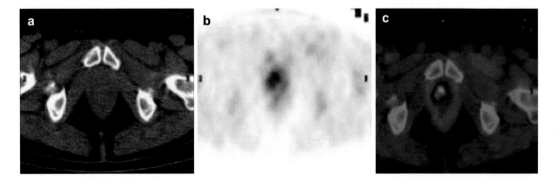

This 71-year-old man (C.B.) was referred for a TRUS-guided biopsy in April 2010 for suspicion of PC. The serum PSA levels at the time of investigation were 18 ng/mL. At TRUS, no pathological area was identified and the gland was considered normal by dimension. A 12-core biopsy did not demonstrate malignant cells. In June 2010, a ^{11}C-choline PET/CT (A low-dose CT, B PET, C fusion images) demonstrated a focus of ^{11}C-choline uptake in the gland apex. A TRUS-guided biopsy was performed, guided by ^{11}C-choline PET/CT, and histological examination of the specimen demonstrated prostate cancer cells (GS = 4+4) in the area of ^{11}C-choline maximum uptake.

Case 5.3

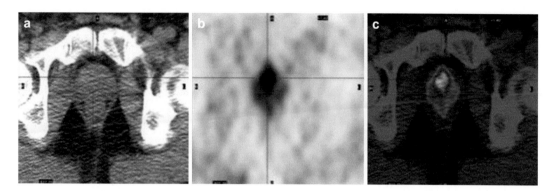

This 63-year-old man (S.R.) was referred for a prostate biopsy because of clinical suspicion of PC with serum PSA levels of 15 ng/mL and after a negative DRE. On April 2010, a 12-core TRUS-guided biopsy was negative. Four weeks later, a ^{11}C-choline PET/CT (A low-dose CT, B PET, C fusion images) demonstrated a focus of intense ^{11}C-choline uptake in the central and anterior part of the gland. On the basis of ^{11}C-choline PET/CT, the patient was referred to a radical prostatectomy. Histological examination of the specimen demonstrated the presence of an inflammatory process (acute prostatitis) but no malignant cells.

Case 5.4

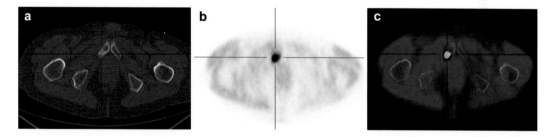

This 60-year-old patient (C.S.) was scheduled for a radical prostatectomy for a proven PC (Gleason score 4 + 3, initial PSA 12.7 ng/mL) on June 2012. On July 2012, a staging ^{11}C-choline PET/CT was performed and showed a diffuse uptake in the central part of the prostate gland (not reported) and an intense focal uptake on the right pubis (A low-dose CT, B PET, C fusion images). A bone biopsy was subsequently performed and confirmed the presence of a PC metastatic lesion. The patient was addressed to a palliative treatment with androgen deprivation therapy and diphosphonate instead a surgery approach.

Case 5.5

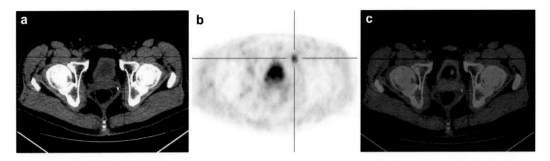

This 68-year-old man (C.R.) was treated on August 2011 with a radical prostatectomy and adjuvant androgen deprivation therapy for a PC (pT3bN0M0; Gleason score 4+4, initial PSA 14.1 ng/mL). PSA nadir after treatment was <0.2 ng/mL. After 22 months from surgery, PSA starts to increase until reaching the value of 1.5 ng/mL (PSA doubling time 5 months, PSA velocity 1.8 ng/mL/year) on December 2012. Three weeks later, a ^{11}C-choline PET/CT (A low-dose CT, B PET, C fusion images) was performed and demonstrated a focus of ^{11}C-choline uptake on a external iliac lymph node. The patient performed later a salvage radiotherapy on prostatic bed (as suggested by nomogram) and enlarged the field of irradiation with a boost on PET-positive lymph node. After salvage treatment, PSA was not measurable with a biochemical relapse-free survival of 6 months at the end of follow-up.

Case 5.6

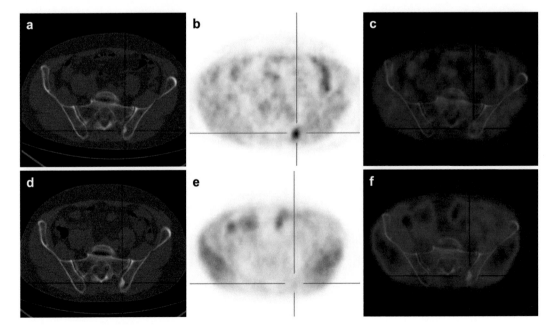

This 7-year-old man (T.F.) was treated on March 2007 with external-beam radiotherapy as the primary treatment for a PC (cT2bN0M0, Gleason score 4 + 3, initial PSA 9.7 ng/mL). On July 2011, PSA raised to 2.5 ng/mL (time to biochemical relapse 52 months), and an LH-RH agonist therapy was administrated. For 6 months, PSA decreased; then on January 2012, PSA raised up to 2.9 ng/mL (PSA doubling time 2 months, PSA velocity 7.2 ng/mL/year) under hormonal therapy. The patient was referred to a ^{11}C-choline PET/CT on February 2012 (A low-dose CT, B PET, C fusion images) that showed a solitary osteoblastic bone lesion on the left ilium. The patient, previously scheduled for a salvage radical prostatectomy according to nomogram, underwent radiotherapy on the solitary lesion and the androgen deprivation therapy scheme was changed. On December 2012, with a PSA of 1.9 ng/mL, a subsequent ^{11}C-choline PET/CT was performed (D low-dose CT, E PET, F fusion images) and showed a metabolic response to the therapy, with no choline uptake on the bone lesion.

References

1. ESMO Guidelines Task Force. ESMO minimum clinical recommendations for diagnosis, treatment and follow-up of prostate cancer. Ann Oncol. 2005;16 Suppl 1:i34–6.
2. Heidenreich A, Bellmunt J, Bolla M, Joniau S, van der Kwast TH, Mason MD, et al. Guidelines on prostate cancer. Eur Urol. 2011;59(4):572–83.
3. Smith RA, Cokkinides V, Eyre HJ. Cancer screening in the United States, 2007: a review of current guidelines, practices, and prospects. CA Cancer J Clin. 2007;57(90):225–49.
4. Mottet N, Bellmunt J, Bolla M, Joniau S, Mason M, Matveev V, et al. EAU guidelines on prostate cancer. Part II: treatment of advanced, relapsing, and castration-resistant prostate cancer. Eur Urol. 2011;59(4):572–83.
5. Phelps ME. Inaugural article: positron emission tomography provides molecular imaging of biological processes. Proc Natl Acad Sci U S A. 2000;97: 9226–33.
6. Sandblom G, Sorensen J, Lundin N, Haggman M, Malmstrom PU. Positron patients with prostate-specific antigen relapse after radical prostatectomy. Urology. 2006;67:996–1000.
7. Dehdashti F, Picus J, Michalski JM, Dence CS, Siegel BA, Katzenellenbogen JA, Welch MJ. Positron tomographic assessment of androgen receptors in prostatic carcinoma. Eur J Nucl Med Mol Imaging. 2005; 32:344–50.
8. Tóth G, Lengyel Z, Balkay L, Salah MA, Trón L, Tóth C. Detection of prostate cancer with 11C-methionine positron emission tomography. J Urol. 2005;173:66–9.
9. Maecke HR, Hofmann M, Haberkorn U. (68) Ga-labeled peptides in tumor imaging. J Nucl Med. 2005;46 Suppl 1:172S–8.
10. Zeisel SH. Dietary choline: biochemistry, physiology and pharmacology. Annu Rev Nutr. 1981;1:95–121.
11. Müller SA, Holzapfel K, Seidl C, Treiber U, Krause BJ, Senekowitsch-Schmidtke R. Characterization of choline uptake in prostate cancer cells following bicalutamide and docetaxel treatment. Eur J Nucl Med Mol Imaging. 2000;36(9):1434–42.
12. Husarik DB, Miralbell R, Dubs M, John H, Giger OT, Gelet A, Cservenyàk T, Hany TF. Evaluation of [(18) F]-choline PET/CT for staging and restaging of prostate cancer. Eur J Nucl Med Mol Imaging. 2008; 35(2):253–63.
13. Mueller-Liesse UG, Miller K. Imaging modalities for primary diagnosis and staging of prostate cancer. Urologe A. 2010;49(2):190–8.
14. Ohori M, Kattan MW, Utsunomiya T, Suyama K, Scardino PT, Wheeler TM. Do impalpable (T1c) cancers visible on ultrasound differ from those not visible? J Urol. 2003;169:964–8.
15. Cornud F, Hamida K, Flam T, Hélénon O, Chrétien Y, Thiounn N, Correas JM, Casanova JM, Moreau JF. Endorectal color doppler sonography and endorectal MR imaging features of nonpalpable prostate cancer: correlation with radical prostatectomy findings. AJR Am J Roentgenol. 2000;175:1161–8.
16. Halpern EJ, Frauscher F, Strup SE, Nazarian LN, O'Kane P, Gomella LG. Prostate: high-frequency Doppler US imaging for cancer detection. Radiology. 2002;225:71–7.
17. Sedelaar JP, Vijverberg PL, De Reijke TM, et al. Transrectal ultrasound in the diagnosis of prostate cancer: state of the art and perspectives. Eur Urol. 2001;40:275–84.
18. Chang JJ, Shinohara K, Bhargava V, et al. Prospective evaluation of lateral biopsies of the peripheral zone for prostate cancer detection. J Urol. 1998;160: 2111–4.
19. Beerlage HP, De Reijke TM, de la Rosette JJ. Considerations regarding prostate biopsies. Eur Urol. 1998;34:303–12.
20. Akin O, Sala E, Moskowitz CS, Kuroiwa K, Ishill NM, Pucar D, Scardino PT, Hricak H. Transition zone prostate cancers: features, detection, localization, and staging at endorectal MR imaging. Radiology. 2006;239:784–92.
21. Engelbrecht MR, Huisman HJ, Laheij RJ, Jager GJ, van Leenders GJ, Hulsbergen-Van DE Kaa CA, de la Rosette JJ, Bickman JG, Barentsz JO. Discrimination

of prostate cancer from normal peripheral zone and central gland tissue by using dynamic contrast-enhanced MR imaging. Radiology. 2003;229:248–54.

22. Buckley DL, Roberts C, Parker GJ, Logue JP, Hutchinson CE. Prostate cancer: evaluation of vascular characteristics with dynamic contrast-enhanced T1-weighted MR imaging—initial experience. Radiology. 2004;233:709–15.

23. Ikonen S, Kivisaari L, Vehmas T, Tervahartiala P, Salo JO, Taari K, Rannikko S. Optimal timing of post-biopsy MR imaging of the prostate. Acta Radiol. 2001;42:70–3.

24. Qayyum A, Coakley FV, Lu Y, Olpin JD, Wu L, Yeh BM, Carroll PR, Kurhanewicz J. Organ confined prostate cancer: effect of prior transrectal biopsy on endorectal MRI and MR spectroscopic imaging. AJR Am J Roentgenol. 2004;183:1079–83.

25. Farsad M, Schwarzenböck S, Krause BJ. PET/CT and choline: diagnosis and staging. Q J Nucl Med Mol Imaging. 2012;56(4):343–53.

26. De Jong JJ, Prium J, Elsinga PH, Vaalburg W, Mensink HJ. 11C-Choline positron emission tomography for the evaluation after treatment of localized prostate cancer. Eur Urol. 2003;44(32):32–8; discussion 8–9.

27. Farsad M, Schiavina R, Castellucci P, Nanni C, Corti B, Martorana G, Canini R, Grigioni W, Boschi S, Marengo M, Pettinato C, Salizzoni E, Monetti N, Franchi R, Fanti S. Detection and localization of prostate cancer: correlation of (11)C-choline PET/CT with histopathologic step-section analysis. J Nucl Med. 2005;46:1642–9.

28. Reske SN, Blumstein NM, Neumaier B, Gottfried HW, Finsterbusch F, Kocot D, Moller P, Glatting G, Perner S. Imaging prostate cancer with 11C-choline PET/CT. J Nucl Med. 2006;47:1249–54.

29. Giovacchini G, Picchio M, Coradeschi E, Scattoni V, Bettinardi C, Cozzarini V, et al. [(11)C]choline uptake with PET/CT for the initial diagnosis of prostate cancer: relation to PSA levels, tumour stage and anti-androgenic therapy. Eur J Nucl Med Mol Imaging. 2008;35:1065–73.

30. Martorana G, Schiavina R, Corti B, Farsad M, Salizzoni E, Brunocilla E, Bertaccini A, Manferrari F, Castellucci P, Fanti S, Canini R, Grigioni WF, D'Errico Grigioni A. 11C-choline positron emission tomography/computerized tomography for tumor localization of primary prostate cancer in comparison with 12-core biopsy. J Urol. 2006;176:954–60.

31. Testa C, Schiavina R, Lodi R, Salizzoni E, Corti B, Farsad M, et al. Prostate cancer: sextant localization with MR imaging, MR spectroscopy, and 11C-choline PET/CT. Radiology. 2007;244(3):797–806. Epub 2007 Jul 24.

FLT PET/CT-Guided Biopsy in the Evaluation of Cancer

Lucia Zanoni, Andreas K. Buck, and Ken Herrmann

6.1 ^{18}F-FLT PET/CT for Evaluation of Solid Tumors

Deregulated cell cycle progression is a hallmark of cancer [1, 2]. The majority of therapeutic drugs have been designed to inhibit cell proliferation and/or to induce apoptosis. Metabolic imaging with positron emission tomography (PET) and the glucose analog 2′-[18F]fluoro-2′-deoxyglucose (^{18}F-FDG) is a sensitive imaging modality to detect malignant tumors and to identify response to therapy early in the course of anticancer treatment [3, 4].^{18}F-FDG is also a valuable clinical tool for predicting tumor response to therapy and patient survival [5, 6]. However, tumoral uptake of ^{18}F-FDG is a bio-

marker of glucose metabolism and is associated with false positive findings in inflammatory processes [7, 8].

Therefore, other tracers that complement the information provided by ^{18}F-FDG have been investigated. Several DNA precursors have been investigated as biomarker of cellular proliferation, including ^{11}C-thymidine which represents the native pyrimidine base used for DNA synthesis in vivo [9]. Due to the short half-life of ^{11}C and rapid degradation of ^{11}C-thymidine, this tracer is not practical for clinical use.

^{18}F-fluoro-3-deoxy-3-L-fluorothymidine (^{18}F-FLT) has been developed as a surrogate PET marker of cellular proliferation [10]. Being a key component of tumor development and growth, cell proliferation is an attractive biological target in cancer imaging. ^{18}F-FLT uptake is independent from glucose metabolism: thymidine is a native nucleoside which is utilized by proliferating cells for DNA replication during the S-phase of the cell cycle. ^{18}F-FLT is handled by the cytosolic thymidine kinase 1 (TK1), the salvage pathway key enzyme, whose activity is cell cycle dependent and three to four times higher in malignant cells than in benign cells. In vitro studies indicated excellent correlation between ^{18}F-FLT uptake and the amount of cells in S-phase of the cell cycle, TK1 overexpression or Ki-67 expression [11]. At present, cellular proliferation can be assessed only by a number of in vitro assays performed in biopsy-derived tissue specimens.

L. Zanoni (✉)
Department of Nuclear Medicine, University Hospital Sant'Orsola-Malpighi, Bologna, Italy
e-mail: luciaironic@hotmail.it;
lucia.zanoni@aosp.bo.it

A.K. Buck
Department of Nuclear Medicine, University of Würzburg, Würzburg, Germany
e-mail: Buck_A@ukw.de

K. Herrmann
Department of Nuclear Medicine, University of Würzburg, Würzburg, Germany

Ahmanson Translational Imaging Division, Department of Molecular and Medical Pharmacology, David Geffen School of Medicine at UCLA, Los Angeles, CA, USA
e-mail: herrmann_k1@ukw.de

© Springer International Publishing 2016
J. Cerci et al. (eds.), *Oncological PET/CT with Histological Confirmation*,
DOI 10.1007/978-3-319-27880-3_6

However, biopsy may be difficult depending on the location of the tumor. Moreover, due to tumor heterogeneity, biopsy results may not be representative of the proliferating activity of the whole tumor or metastatic sites. In addition, excisional biopsy is associated with complications making a full surgical procedure necessary, i.e., in case of mediastinal or intra-abdominal tumors or patients who underwent radiotherapy [12].

Studies in patients revealed high bone marrow uptake and significant tracer retention in the liver and the urinary tract, including the kidneys and bladder. This observation is related to the clearance route of ^{18}F-FLT which is excreted in a nonmetabolized form. In terms of radiation exposure, ^{18}F-FLT produces similar whole-body and bladder wall radiation doses, as compared to ^{18}F-FDG. The brain and heart receive lower doses, while the liver and bone marrow receive higher doses compared to ^{18}F-FDG. All the studies comparing ^{18}F-FLT to ^{18}F-FDG retention in tumor tissue demonstrated that the ^{18}F-FDG SUVmax was significantly higher than that of ^{18}F-FLT. Despite this limitation, ^{18}F-FLT uptake in the surrounding tissue was proven to be low. Therefore, tumor/normal tissue ratios of ^{18}F-FLT are similar to that of ^{18}F-FDG, thus enabling good visualization of ^{18}F-FLT-positive lesions [13–15]. ^{18}F-FLT has already been successfully used to study solid malignancies, and preliminary results confirmed the capability of this tracer to discriminate cancer from inflammation. This has been shown in patients with pancreatic [16] or lung lesions [17]. In numerous tumors, a good correlation was found between ^{18}F-FLT SUV and cancer proliferative activity, as determined by Ki-67 or proliferating cell nuclear antigen (PCNA) immunostaining of resected tissue specimens [18, 19].

Proliferation markers should not be considered as replacement of ^{18}F-FDG but rather as complementary, providing additional information on the proliferative activity of tumors. This information could be used to improve the specificity of noninvasive imaging and better discrimination of viable tumor and necrotic or scar tissue. Furthermore, ^{18}F-FLT PET could serve as a diagnostic tool to noninvasively assess the tumor grade in all sites of the tumor and to visualize intra-lesional and inter-lesional heterogeneity and as a guide to the optimum site for biopsy. The higher specificity of ^{18}F-FLT, as compared to ^{18}F-FDG, may contribute to select those patients who might benefit from adjuvant treatment or from tailored therapeutic regimens [20–22].

Measuring tumor proliferative activity with ^{18}F-FLT PET offers great potential for assessing the viability of tumor cells during or early after treatment because ^{18}F-FLT uptake suppression occurs far before treatment-induced change in tumor size becomes measurable. For ^{18}F-FDG it has also been shown that the proliferation rate significantly contributes to the tumor uptake of the radiotracer [23–25]. However, preclinical and clinical comparison studies showed that ^{18}F-FLT uptake better correlates with proliferation indexes than ^{18}F-FDG [17, 26]. Furthermore, ^{18}F-FDG can better discriminate viable tumor from scar tissue and can detect response to treatment very early in the course of treatment [5]. Recently, the accuracy of posttreatment or interim FDG-PET studies has been questioned due to a reduced specificity of ^{18}F-FDG [27], caused by tracer uptake in inflammatory lesions. In preclinical and clinical studies, higher sensitivity and specificity of ^{18}F-FLT as compared to ^{18}F-FDG has been reported [28–30]. Whether the higher accuracy of ^{18}F-FLT over ^{18}F-FDG holds up also in future clinical studies remains to be determined.

Moreover, ^{18}F-FLT uptake and retention within the tumor cells is directed by a variety of not yet clearly defined factors. The most probable factors currently discussed include loss of cell cycle control, resulting from gain of function of oncogenes, loss of function of tumor suppressor genes, and genome maintenance genes [15]. Although cellular proliferation is a hallmark of malignancy, an increased rate of cell division can also occur in benign processes. High ^{18}F-FLT uptake in nonmetastatic lymph nodes was proven to be related to reactive B-lymphocyte proliferation in the germinal center. In addition, increased perfusion and vascular permeability, not only proliferation of inflammatory cells, can result in nonspecific ^{18}F-FLT uptake in benign lesions [31].

A systematic review and meta-analysis of 27 different studies (1998–2011) with a total of 509 patients was performed by the London group of Chalkidou and co-workers [18]. The authors showed that, given an appropriate study design, the ^{18}F-FLT /Ki-67 correlation is significant and independent of cancer type with either the use of Ki-67 average measurement regardless of the nature of the sample or whole surgical samples when measuring Ki-67 maximum expression. In particular, there are already sufficient data to support a strong correlation for brain, lung, and breast cancer [18].

The following six cases will show the normal distribution of ^{18}F-FLT, likely future indications including lung cancer [17], sarcoma [32], gastric cancer [33], brain malignancies [34, 35], pancreatic cancer [16, 36], and lymphoma [37, 38].

6.2 ^{18}F-FLT PET/CT for Evaluation of Lymphoma

As ^{18}F-FDG already provides a very sensitive imaging tool for detection of lymphoma [39], ^{18}F-FLT should not be regarded as an alternative to the ^{18}F-FDG but rather as an imaging biomarker providing complementary information. As there is high uptake of ^{18}F-FLT in normal bone marrow, ^{18}F-FLT is not useful for evaluation of marrow involvement by lymphoma. In addition given its lower tumor-to-normal tissue contrast, the clinical usefulness of ^{18}F-FLT PET for staging lymphoma is likely limited due to the low tumor-to-normal tissue ratio of uptake compared to ^{18}F-FDG. The only advantages of ^{18}F-FLT could be for detection of lymphoma in the central nervous system (CNS) and in the mediastinum [40].

Besides tumor detection and assessment of proliferation, ^{18}F-FLT PET has been shown to differentiate between high- and low-grade lymphoma (a suitable cutoff value of SUV = 3 was described). Variants of lymphoma with low mitotic indices would be expected to have low ^{18}F-FLT avidity, and indolent lymphomas are likely to have lower ^{18}F-FLT uptake than aggressive ones, based on differences in genomic expression related to cell cycling [41].

In animal studies a decrease in ^{18}F-FLT uptake can be detected as early as 24 h after chemotherapy, preceding a change of tumor volume at a later time point; it correlates well with cell cycle arrest and it is inversely correlated to induction of apoptosis as demonstrated by immunohistochemical studies [42].

For both murine lymphoma xenotransplant models and human high-grade non-Hodgkin lymphoma (NHL), chemotherapy is associated with an early decrease in lymphoma ^{18}F-FLT uptake. Interestingly it happens with R-CHOP/CHOP administration (R = rituximab; CHOP = cyclophosphamide, doxorubicin, vincristine, and prednisone) but not with rituximab alone, indicating no early antiproliferative effect of immunotherapy [37].

A rapid decline in ^{18}F-FLT uptake after 1 week of therapy was also noted in patients affected by mantle cell lymphoma [43]. More attention has been recently paid to prognostic implications of ^{18}F-FLT uptake.

High initial ^{18}F-FLT uptake correlates with IPI score and is a negative predictor of response to R-CHOP in aggressive NHL, representing a promising tool for implementing risk-adapted treatment in these patients [44]. Kasper and collaborators assessed both ^{18}F-FDG and ^{18}F-FLT in the restaging of 48 lymphoma patients with residual masses greater than 2 cm in diameter [38]. Patients in whom both ^{18}F-FDG and ^{18}F-FLT were positive had an extremely poor survival (less than 1 year); patients in whom both the scans were negative did not relapse nor die during a surveillance range of 4–32 months. However, it is not practical, nor cost-effective, to use both tracers routinely. ^{18}F-FLT may help to select which patients with a positive post-treatment ^{18}F-FDG PET require more aggressive investigation or therapy. A negative ^{18}F-FLT scan may allow ongoing surveillance, and a positive ^{18}F-FLT scan may identify those patients requiring treatment intensification [38].

According to a recent Chinese study by a group from Beijing, it seems more objective to use the SUVmax ratio (tumor to mediastinum) rather than SUVmax alone for the uptake measurements [45].

Cases 4, 5, and 6 illustrate the role of ^{18}F-FLT PET/CT in patients with lymphoma presenting with positive or equivocal ^{18}F-FDG findings after treatment or during the follow-up evaluation. The theoretical application of ^{18}F-FLT PET/CT in the particular subset of patients with a suspect of residual or recurrent disease is aimed to identify early relapse. However, further studies are needed to investigate possible false-positive results with ^{18}F-FLT.

Case 6.1
Patient with non-small-cell lung cancer (NSCLC) (Adapted from Buck et al. [17]).

A 75-year-old male with NSCLC in the left upper lobe underwent ^{18}F-FLT PET and ^{18}F-FDG PET for tumor staging. Transaxial ^{18}F-FLT PET demonstrates physiologic tracer uptake in the bone marrow compartment including the vertebral

column, scapula, and ribs (Fig. 6.1a). ^{18}F-FLT uptake can also be seen in the margin of the primary lung tumor (arrow). The corresponding ^{18}F-FDG PET scan (Fig. 6.1b) shows also high ^{18}F-FDG uptake at the tumor margin of the lung tumor. Figure 6.1c displays the corresponding CT scan with the lung mass (arrow). Immunostaining of the resected tumor demonstrates a high proliferation rate of 54 % (Fig. 6.1d).

In this study, it was shown that ^{18}F-FLT uptake correlates better with proliferation of lung tumors than uptake of ^{18}F-FDG [17]. In an additional study, it was shown that FLT-PET has a high specificity for the detection of malignant lung tumors. However, compared to ^{18}F-FDG, ^{18}F-FLT PET was inferior for N- and M-staging [46]. Therefore, it was concluded that ^{18}F-FLT PET cannot be recommended for staging of lung cancer.

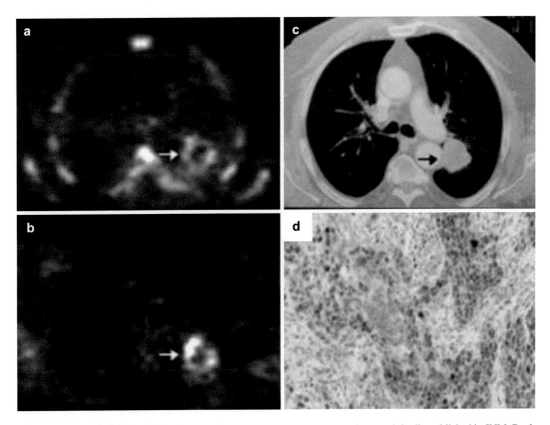

Fig. 6.1 Patient with non-small-cell lung cancer (staging) including transaxial ^{18}F-FLT (**a**), ^{18}F-FDG (**b**), and computed tomography (**c**) images and immunostaining (**d**) (This research was originally published in JNM. Buck et al. [17] © by the Society of Nuclear Medicine and Molecular Imaging, Inc.)

Case 6.2

Patient with sarcoma (Modified according to Buck et al. [32]).

A 34-year-old woman with a primary low-grade soft tissue sarcoma of the left distal thigh underwent ^{18}F-FDG PET/CT for staging. Corresponding maximum intensity projection is shown in Fig. 6.2a, revealing intense tracer uptake in the malignant primary and in pulmonary metastases (Fig. 6.2e and f). An additional ^{18}F-FLT PET scan (maximum intensity projection, Fig. 6.2b) was performed, showing only faint ^{18}F-FLT uptake in the primary lesion (mean ^{18}F-FLT SUVmean: 1.0, Fig. 6.2c). Interestingly, the lung lesions showed mild to moderate ^{18}F-FLT uptake with a mean ^{18}F-FLT SUVmean of up to 2.2 (Fig. 6.2d). Corresponding sections of helical CT show the primary tumor (Fig. 6.2g)

and large pulmonary metastases in both lungs (Fig. 6.2h, arrows).

As part of the clinical work-up, the primary tumor and a lung metastasis were biopsied. Corresponding anti-Ki-67 immunostaining (MIB1) of tissue derived from the primary tumor in the left thigh indicates a low proliferation fraction (<5 % brown-labeled nuclei; Fig. 6.2i) in agreement with only faint ^{18}F-FLT uptake (Fig. 6.2c). In contrast, the Ki-67 immunohistochemistry of a pulmonary metastasis indicates higher proliferative activity (15 % proliferating cells, Fig. 6.2j) and was assigned grade 2, also in agreement with the mild to moderate ^{18}F-FLT uptake (Fig. 6.2d).

This representative case documents the superiority of ^{18}F-FLT PET for differentiation of low- and high-grade sarcomas as previously shown in 15 patients [32].

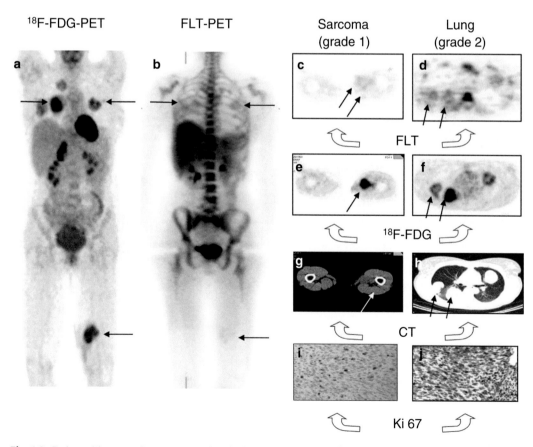

Fig. 6.2 Patient with metastatic sarcoma (staging) including maximum intensity projection (MIP) of ^{18}F-FDG PET (**a**) and ^{18}F-FLT PET (**b**). Corresponding transaxial images are shown for ^{18}F-FLT PET (**c, d**), for ^{18}F-FDG PET (**e, f**), and for CT (**g, h**). Immunostainings for the primary tumor (**i**) and the lung metastasis (**j**) are also shown

Case 6.3

18F-FLT PET in a patient with hepatocellular carcinoma (Modified from Eckel et al. [47]).

A 58-year-old male patient with biopsy-proven multifocal hepatocellular cancer underwent ^{18}F-FLT PET. Coronal (Fig. 6.3a) and transaxial (Fig. 6.3b) images are displayed, revealing an intense ^{18}F-FLT uptake in projection of one of the multifocal tumor manifestations. The corresponding SUVmean and SUVmax were 11.1 and 14.3, respectively. Given the liver uptake values of 4.8 and 5.9 for SUVmean and SUVmax, this tumor was rated as visually positive. Figures 6.3c and d display the corresponding axial MRI.

Hematoxylin-eosin staining with a 20-fold magnification is shown in Fig. 6.3e. The corresponding immunostaining is displayed in Fig. 6.3f with a proliferative activity of 30 %.

Despite the high physiologic liver uptake, this study showed a sensitivity of 69 % for detection of hepatocellular carcinoma with ^{18}F-FLT PET. This pilot trial also demonstrated that a high initial ^{18}F-FLT uptake was associated with a reduced overall survival underlining the prognostic potential of ^{18}F-FLT PET [47].

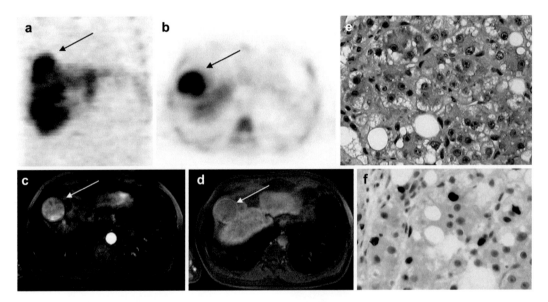

Fig. 6.3 Patient with metastatic hepatocellular cancer (staging) including coronal (**a**) and transaxial (**b**) ^{18}F-FLT PET, corresponding MRI images (**c**, **d**), hematoxylin-eosin staining (**e**, magnification × 20), and immunostaining for MIB1 (**f**, magnification × 20) (This research was originally published in JNM. Eckel et al. [47] © by the Society of Nuclear Medicine and Molecular Imaging, Inc.)

Case 6.4

Anaplastic large T-cell lymphoma relapse with *¹⁸F-FDG and ¹⁸F-FLT-avid cervical and groin* *lymphadenopathy.*

A 60-year-old man was diagnosed with non-Hodgkin anaplastic large T-cell lymphoma (ALCL) (ALK negative) (stage IIIA, IPI 1) in August 2011. He was first treated with 12 cycles of MACOP-B (methotrexate, doxorubicin, cyclophosphamide, vincristine, prednisone, and bleomycin). The end-treatment ¹⁸F-FDG PET/CT demonstrated an avid cervical lymphadenopathy. Due to first-line treatment failure, the patient received two cycles of IEV chemotherapy (ifosfamide, epirubicin, and etoposide), achieving a complete meta-

bolic response (at the pre-transplant evaluation with ¹⁸F-FDG PET). An autologous stem cell transplant was performed in July 2012. In January 2013, he presented with clinical suspicions of relapse, and a follow-up ¹⁸F-FDG PET/CT showed at least two new ¹⁸F-FDG-avid lymph nodes in the left groin (SUVmax of 9 and the maximum diameter was 22 mm) and the reappearance of some other avid lymph nodes in the right neck (SUVmax of 10). ¹⁸F-FLT PET/CT performed 2 weeks later confirmed all previous findings, showing high uptake in the left groin (SUVmax of 14) and right neck (SUVmax of 16.8). A biopsy of the left groin confirmed the presence of ALCL relapse (Fig. 6.4a and b).

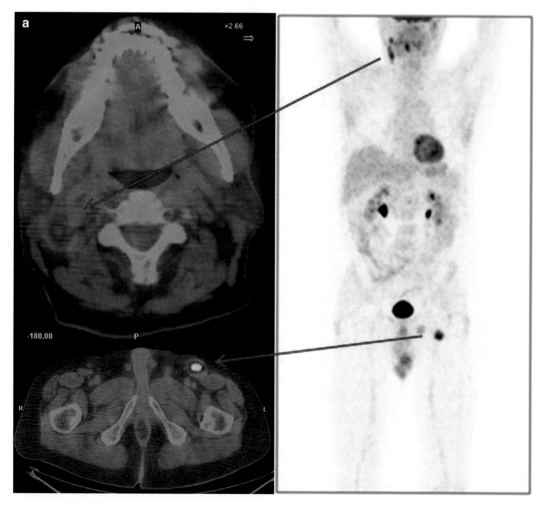

Fig. 6.4 (a) ¹⁸F-FDG-avid cervical and groin lymphadenopathy (*arrows*) (*left*, transaxial fused images; *right*, MIP). (b) Same cervical and groin lymphadenopathy showing intense ¹⁸F-FLT uptake (*arrows*) (*left*, transaxial fused images; *right*, MIP)

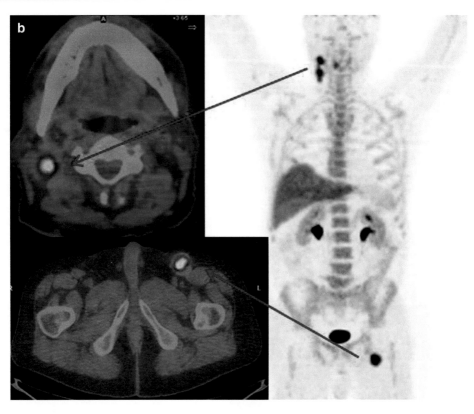

Fig. 6.4 (continued)

Case 6.5

Recurrent mantle cell lymphoma of the bowel (Ki-67/MIB1: 30 %) with ^{18}F-FDG and ^{18}F-FLT-avid supra- and subdiaphragmatic lymphadenopathy and bowel involvement

A 65-year-old woman was diagnosed with mantle cell NHL (stage I, with gastric and bowel involvement) in 2011. She was first treated with RFN (rituximab, fludarabine, and novantrone), achieving a complete metabolic response. In September 2012, relapse was suspected although a biopsy of the right groin and of the stomach showed only inflammatory cells. In March 2013, ^{18}F-FDG PET/CT showed increased uptake in multiple left axillary nodes (SUVmax of 5 versus previous of 3.4); new ^{18}F-FDG-avid right axillary, right paratracheal (SUVmax of 9.6) and superior phrenic (SUVmax of 7.5) retroperitoneal; and mesenteric nodes near the cecum (SUVmax of 9.4). In addition there was diffuse intense uptake all along the bowel, more prominent at the level of the right and transverse colon, and some small-bowel loops, which appeared dilated in the corresponding low-dose CT images. Focal uptake was found in the right iliac fossa (SUVmax of 11.6). The known groin lymph nodes disappeared. All these findings were highly suspicious for relapse of lymphoma. The same lesions were ^{18}F-FLT avid on a scan performed approximately 20 days later: ^{18}F- SUVmax of 5.5 left axillary, 9.3 right paratracheal, 7.2 superior phrenic, 9.3 cecum area, and 9.2 at the level of the bowel in the right iliac fossa. Histological examination of an endoscopic biopsy at the level of the iliac-cecum junction demonstrated mantle cell lymphoma (CD20−, CD79+, and BCL1+ at IHC) with a proliferative index of 30 % measured by Ki-67/MIB1. The bone marrow biopsy was positive with 20 % cellularity. The patient underwent second-line therapy for recurrent disease (Fig. 6.5).

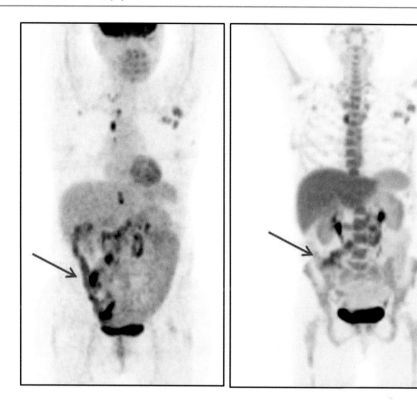

Fig. 6.5 Comparison of ^{18}F-FDG (*left*) and ^{18}F-FLT (*right*) showing avid supra- and subdiaphragmatic nodes and diffuse uptake in the bowel, more focal in the right iliac fossa (*arrows*)

Case 6.6

Follicular lymphoma relapse (MIB1 70 %): ^{18}F-FDG and ^{18}F-FLT-avid subdiaphragmatic lymphadenopathy

A 43-year-old woman was diagnosed with grade II/IIIA follicular lymphoma (stage IV with bone marrow involvement) in November 2009. She was treated with six cycles of R-CHOP chemotherapy.

The follow-up ^{18}F-FDG PET/CT revealed the presence of multiple avid bilateral external iliac, bilateral obturator, and right groin lymphadenopathy (SUVmax of 5). ^{18}F-FLT PET/CT showed moderate uptake at the level of the previous findings (SUVmax of 5.6 external iliac, 3.9 internal iliac, and 4.5 right groin). Relapse of follicular lymphoma was confirmed by histological examination of the right groin lymphadenopathy. The proliferation index measured by MIB1 was 70 %. The bone marrow biopsy was positive; ^{18}F-FDG follow-up scan performed a few months later showed progressive disease with both supra- and mainly subdiaphragmatic lesions. The patient underwent second-line therapy leading to remission (Fig. 6.6a and b).

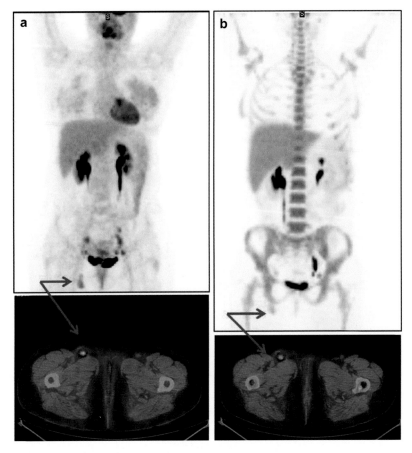

Fig. 6.6 (**a**) ^{18}F-FDG-avid right groin lymphadenopathy (*arrows*) (*lower*, transaxial fused image; *upper*, MIP). (**b**) The same right groin lymphadenopathy showing intense ^{18}F-FLT uptake (*arrows*) (*lower*, transaxial fused image; *upper*, MIP)

References

1. Hanahan D, Weinberg RA. Hallmarks of cancer: the next generation. Cell. 2011;144(5):646–74.
2. Hanahan D, Weinberg RA. The hallmarks of cancer. Cell. 2000;100(1):57–70.
3. Barentsz J, Takahashi S, Oyen W, Mus R, De Mulder P, Reznek R, Oudkerk M, Mali W. Commonly used imaging techniques for diagnosis and staging. J Clin Oncol. 2006;24(20):3234–44.
4. von Schulthess GK, Steinert HC, Hany TF. Integrated PET/CT: current applications and future directions. Radiology. 2006;238(2):405–22.
5. Herrmann K, Benz MR, Krause BJ, Pomykala KL, Buck AK, Czernin J. (18)F-FDG-PET/CT in evaluating response to therapy in solid tumors: where we are and where we can go. Q J Nucl Med Mol Imaging. 2011;55(6):620–32.
6. Juweid ME, Cheson BD. Positron-emission tomography and assessment of cancer therapy. N Engl J Med. 2006;354(5):496–507.
7. Kubota R, Kubota K, Yamada S, Tada M, Ido T, Tamahashi N. Microautoradiographic study for the differentiation of intratumoral macrophages, granulation tissues and cancer cells by the dynamics of fluorine-18-fluorodeoxyglucose uptake. J Nucl Med. 1994;35(1):104–12.
8. Shreve PD, Anzai Y, Wahl RL. Pitfalls in oncologic diagnosis with FDG PET imaging: physiologic and benign variants. Radiographics. 1999;19(1):61–77. quiz 150–151.
9. Wells P, Gunn RN, Alison M, Steel C, Golding M, Ranicar AS, Brady F, Osman S, Jones T, Price P. Assessment of proliferation in vivo using 2-[(11)C]thymidine positron emission tomography in advanced intra-abdominal malignancies. Cancer Res. 2002;62(20):5698–702.
10. Shields AF, Grierson JR, Dohmen BM, Machulla HJ, Stayanoff JC, Lawhorn-Crews JM, Obradovich JE, Muzik O, Mangner TJ. Imaging proliferation in vivo with [F-18]FLT and positron emission tomography. Nat Med. 1998;4(11):1334–6.

11. Salskov A, Tammisetti VS, Grierson J, Vesselle H. FLT: measuring tumor cell proliferation in vivo with positron emission tomography and 3′-deoxy-3′-[18F]fluorothymidine. Semin Nucl Med. 2007;37(6): 429–39.

12. Mankoff DA, Shields AF, Krohn KA. PET imaging of cellular proliferation. Radiol Clin North Am. 2005;43(1):153–67.

13. Bading JR, Shields AF. Imaging of cell proliferation: status and prospects. J Nucl Med. 2008;49 Suppl 2:64S–80.

14. Been LB, Suurmeijer AJ, Cobben DC, Jager PL, Hoekstra HJ, Elsinga PH. [18F]FLT-PET in oncology: current status and opportunities. Eur J Nucl Med Mol Imaging. 2004;31(12):1659–72.

15. Buck AK, Herrmann K, Shen C, Dechow T, Schwaiger M, Wester HJ. Molecular imaging of proliferation in vivo: positron emission tomography with [18F]fluorothymidine. Methods. 2009;48(2):205–15.

16. Herrmann K, Eckel F, Schmidt S, Scheidhauer K, Krause BJ, Kleeff J, Schuster T, Wester HJ, Friess H, Schmid RM, et al. In vivo characterization of proliferation for discriminating cancer from pancreatic pseudotumors. J Nucl Med. 2008;49(9):1437–44.

17. Buck AK, Halter G, Schirrmeister H, Kotzerke J, Wurziger I, Glatting G, Mattfeldt T, Neumaier B, Reske SN, Hetzel M. Imaging proliferation in lung tumors with PET: 18F-FLT versus 18F-FDG. J Nucl Med. 2003;44(9):1426–31.

18. Chalkidou A, Landau DB, Odell EW, Cornelius VR, O'Doherty MJ, Marsden PK. Correlation between Ki-67 immunohistochemistry and 18F-fluorothymidine uptake in patients with cancer: a systematic review and meta-analysis. Eur J Cancer. 2012;48(18):3499–513.

19. van Waarde A, Elsinga PH. Proliferation markers for the differential diagnosis of tumor and inflammation. Curr Pharm Des. 2008;14(31):3326–39.

20. Barwick T, Bencherif B, Mountz JM, Avril N. Molecular PET and PET/CT imaging of tumour cell proliferation using F-18 fluoro-L-thymidine: a comprehensive evaluation. Nucl Med Commun. 2009;30(12):908–17.

21. Shields AF. Positron emission tomography measurement of tumor metabolism and growth: its expanding role in oncology. Mol Imaging Biol. 2006;8(3): 141–50.

22. Tehrani OS, Shields AF. PET imaging of proliferation with pyrimidines. J Nucl Med. 2013;54(6):903–12.

23. Bos R, van Der Hoeven JJ, van Der Wall E, van Der Groep P, van Diest PJ, Comans EF, Joshi U, Semenza GL, Hoekstra OS, Lammertsma AA, et al. Biologic correlates of (18)fluorodeoxyglucose uptake in human breast cancer measured by positron emission tomography. J Clin Oncol. 2002;20(2):379–87.

24. Buck AK, Schirrmeister H, Mattfeldt T, Reske SN. Biological characterisation of breast cancer by means of PET. Eur J Nucl Med Mol Imaging. 2004;31 Suppl 1:S80–7.

25. Higashi K, Clavo AC, Wahl RL. Does FDG uptake measure proliferative activity of human cancer cells? In vitro comparison with DNA flow cytometry and tritiated thymidine uptake. J Nucl Med. 1993; 34(3):414–9.

26. Vesselle H, Grierson J, Muzi M, Pugsley JM, Schmidt RA, Rabinowitz P, Peterson LM, Vallieres E, Wood DE. In vivo validation of 3′deoxy-3′-[(18)F]fluorothymidine ([(18)F]FLT) as a proliferation imaging tracer in humans: correlation of [(18)F]FLT uptake by positron emission tomography with Ki-67 immunohistochemistry and flow cytometry in human lung tumors. Clin Cancer Res. 2002;8(11):3315–23.

27. Moskowitz CH, Schoder H, Teruya-Feldstein J, Sima C, Iasonos A, Portlock CS, Straus D, Noy A, Palomba ML, O'Connor OA, et al. Risk-adapted dose-dense immunochemotherapy determined by interim FDG-PET in advanced-stage diffuse large B-Cell lymphoma. J Clin Oncol. 2010;28(11):1896–903.

28. Graf N, Herrmann K, Numberger B, Zwisler D, Aichler M, Feuchtinger A, Schuster T, Wester HJ, Senekowitsch-Schmidtke R, Peschel C, et al. [18F] FLT is superior to [18F]FDG for predicting early response to antiproliferative treatment in high-grade lymphoma in a dose-dependent manner. Eur J Nucl Med Mol Imaging. 2013;40(1):34–43.

29. Leonard JP, LaCasce AS, Smith MR, Noy A, Chirieac LR, Rodig SJ, Yu JQ, Vallabhajosula S, Schoder H, English P, et al. Selective CDK4/6 inhibition with tumor responses by PD0332991 in patients with mantle cell lymphoma. Blood. 2012;119(20):4597–607.

30. Li Z, Graf N, Herrmann K, Junger A, Aichler M, Feuchtinger A, Baumgart A, Walch A, Peschel C, Schwaiger M, et al. FLT-PET is superior to FDG-PET for very early response prediction in NPM-ALK-positive lymphoma treated with targeted therapy. Cancer Res. 2012;72(19):5014–24.

31. Troost EG, Vogel WV, Merkx MA, Slootweg PJ, Marres HA, Peeters WJ, Bussink J, van der Kogel AJ, Oyen WJ, Kaanders JH. 18F-FLT PET does not discriminate between reactive and metastatic lymph nodes in primary head and neck cancer patients. J Nucl Med. 2007;48(5):726–35.

32. Buck AK, Herrmann K, Buschenfelde CM, Juweid ME, Bischoff M, Glatting G, Weirich G, Moller P, Wester HJ, Scheidhauer K, et al. Imaging bone and soft tissue tumors with the proliferation marker [18F] fluorodeoxythymidine. Clin Cancer Res. 2008;14(10): 2970–7.

33. Herrmann K, Ott K, Buck AK, Lordick F, Wilhelm D, Souvatzoglou M, Becker K, Schuster T, Wester HJ, Siewert JR, et al. Imaging gastric cancer with PET and the radiotracers 18F-FLT and 18F-FDG: a comparative analysis. J Nucl Med. 2007;48(12):1945–50.

34. Chen W, Cloughesy T, Kamdar N, Satyamurthy N, Bergsneider M, Liau L, Mischel P, Czernin J, Phelps ME, Silverman DH. Imaging proliferation in brain tumors with 18F-FLT PET: comparison with 18F-FDG. J Nucl Med. 2005;46(6):945–52.

35. Ullrich R, Backes H, Li H, Kracht L, Miletic H, Kesper K, Neumaier B, Heiss WD, Wienhard K, Jacobs AH. Glioma proliferation as assessed by 3′-fluoro-3′-deoxy-L-thymidine positron emission tomography in patients with newly diagnosed high-grade glioma. Clin Cancer Res. 2008;14(7): 2049–55.

36. Herrmann K, Erkan M, Dobritz M, Schuster T, Siveke JT, Beer AJ, Wester HJ, Schmid RM, Friess H, Schwaiger M, et al. Comparison of 3′-deoxy-3′-[(1) (8)F]fluorothymidine positron emission tomography (FLT PET) and FDG PET/CT for the detection and characterization of pancreatic tumours. Eur J Nucl Med Mol Imaging. 2012;39(5):846–51.

37. Herrmann K, Wieder HA, Buck AK, Schoffel M, Krause BJ, Fend F, Schuster T, Meyer zum Buschenfelde C, Wester HJ, Duyster J, et al. Early response assessment using 3′-deoxy-3′-[18F] fluorothymidine-positron emission tomography in high-grade non-Hodgkin's lymphoma. Clin Cancer Res. 2007;13(12):3552–8.

38. Kasper B, Egerer G, Gronkowski M, Haufe S, Lehnert T, Eisenhut M, Mechtersheimer G, Ho AD, Haberkorn U. Functional diagnosis of residual lymphomas after radiochemotherapy with positron emission tomography comparing FDG- and FLT-PET. Leuk Lymphoma. 2007;48(4):746–53.

39. Weiler-Sagie M, Bushelev O, Epelbaum R, Dann EJ, Haim N, Avivi I, Ben-Barak A, Ben-Arie Y, Bar-Shalom R, Israel O. (18)F-FDG avidity in lymphoma readdressed: a study of 766 patients. J Nucl Med. 2010;51(1):25–30.

40. Buchmann I, Neumaier B, Schreckenberger M, Reske S. [18F]3′-deoxy-3′-fluorothymidine-PET in NHL patients: whole-body biodistribution and imaging of lymphoma manifestations--a pilot study. Cancer Biother Radiopharm. 2004;19(4):436–42.

41. Buck AK, Bommer M, Stilgenbauer S, Juweid M, Glatting G, Schirrmeister H, Mattfeldt T, Tepsic D, Bunjes D, Mottaghy FM, et al. Molecular imaging of proliferation in malignant lymphoma. Cancer Res. 2006;66(22):11055–61.

42. Graf N, Herrmann K, den Hollander J, Fend F, Schuster T, Wester HJ, Senekowitsch-Schmidtke R, zum Buschenfelde CM, Peschel C, Schwaiger M, et al. Imaging proliferation to monitor early response of lymphoma to cytotoxic treatment. Mol Imaging Biol. 2008;10(6):349–55.

43. Herrmann K, Buck AK, Schuster T, Rudelius M, Wester HJ, Graf N, Scheuerer C, Peschel C, Schwaiger M, Dechow T, et al. A pilot study to evaluate 3′-deoxy-3′-18F-fluorothymidine pet for initial and early response imaging in mantle cell lymphoma. J Nucl Med. 2011;52(12):1898–902.

44. Herrmann K, Buck AK, Schuster T, Junger A, Wieder HA, Graf N, Ringshausen I, Rudelius M, Wester HJ, Schwaiger M, et al. Predictive value of initial 18F-FLT uptake in patients with aggressive non-Hodgkin lymphoma receiving R-CHOP treatment. J Nucl Med. 2011;52(5):690–6.

45. Wang R, Zhu H, Chen Y, Li C, Li F, Shen Z, Tian J, Yu L, Xu B. Standardized uptake value based evaluation of lymphoma by FDG and FLT PET/CT. Hematol Oncol. 2013;32:126–32.

46. Buck AK, Hetzel M, Schirrmeister H, Halter G, Moller P, Kratochwil C, Wahl A, Glatting G, Mottaghy FM, Mattfeldt T, et al. Clinical relevance of imaging proliferative activity in lung nodules. Eur J Nucl Med Mol Imaging. 2005;32(5):525–33.

47. Eckel F, Herrmann K, Schmidt S, Hillerer C, Wieder HA, Krause BJ, Schuster T, Langer R, Wester HJ, Schmid RM, et al. Imaging of proliferation in hepatocellular carcinoma with the in vivo marker 18F-fluorothymidine. J Nucl Med. 2009;50(9):1441–7.

PET/CT-Guided Biopsy in Pancreatic Lesions

7

Juliano J. Cerci, Mateos Bogoni,
and Dominique Delbeke

7.1   Introduction

Pancreatic cancer represents the fourth most common cause of cancer mortality among men and women worldwide, probably related to its usual delayed diagnosis and aggressive characteristics [1]. The interest in proper evaluation of pancreatic lesions and unveiling their histological aspects has been growing strong over the last years.

The development of image-guided biopsy procedures has also applications for biopsy of the pancreas. Clinical management of potential oncologic patients is greatly facilitated once histological information provided by biopsy is obtained, given that chronic pancreatitis and other benign conditions are possible differential diagnoses of patients suspected of having pancreatic cancer, and implies different therapeutic decisions.

The pancreas is in close anatomic relationship with the stomach and duodenum. Therefore, most pancreatic masses are easily accessible for biopsy with endoscopic ultrasound (EUS). However, endoscopic tissue sampling is limited to fine-needle aspirations. A core biopsy is necessary for histological evaluation. Core biopsies of the pancreas are performed by percutaneous biopsy and are associated with high sensitivity and specificity for malignant tumors [1–3]. In the management of patients with pancreatic cancer, biopsy is not necessary prior to surgery, but as it is essential for neoadjuvant therapy planning, it is usually performed. It is also indicated for staging patients with locally advanced, unresectable cancer or metastatic disease [4].

A direct posterior approach is usually used because of the retroperitoneal location of the pancreas. When a posterior approach is not feasible, solid lesions can be biopsied via a transgastric route [5]. The risk of pancreatitis may be increased when normal pancreatic tissue is included in the biopsy specimen [6].

The imaging modalities used to guide biopsy of the pancreas include not only EUS but also endoscopic cholangioscopy, computerized tomography (CT), magnetic resonance imaging (MRI), and, more recently, positron emission tomography/computerized tomography (PET/CT). CT guidance is the most commonly used procedure for the performance of percutaneous biopsies given its worldwide availability and low rate of complications [7, 8]. However, tumors are heterogeneous and include areas of inflammation and fibrosis, and sampling errors may occur. MRI

J.J. Cerci (✉) • M. Bogoni
Quanta – Diagnóstico e Terapia, Curitiba, PR, Brazil
e-mail: cercijuliano@hotmail.com; bogonimateos@gmail.com

D. Delbeke
Radiology and Radiological Sciences, Vanderbilt University Medical Center, Nashville, TN, USA
e-mail: dominique.delbeke@vanderbilt.edu

© Springer International Publishing 2016
J. Cerci et al. (eds.), *Oncological PET/CT with Histological Confirmation*,
DOI 10.1007/978-3-319-27880-3_7

presents this limitation as well, besides requiring special biopsy instruments, due to the magnetic field created by the scanning process.

In the last 20 years, PET using 2-[18F]-fluoro-2-deoxy-D-glucose (^{18}F-FDG) has become an established modality for metabolic evaluation of oncological patients. The most common clinical application of ^{18}F-FDG PET/CT is initial staging and restaging of ^{18}F-FDG-avid malignancies, including pancreatic cancer [9–11]. However, inflammatory lesions are also ^{18}F-FDG-avid, and biopsy may be necessary for differentiation [12, 13].

In our center, among the 50 patients who underwent ^{18}F-FDG PET/CT for evaluation of a pancreatic lesion and further PET/CT-guided biopsy on the positive cases, 42 were malignant and eight were benign lesions. The sensitivity of the ^{18}F-FDG PET/CT scan was 97.6 % and the specificity was 62.5 %. Similar sensitivity has been reported in the literature for the diagnosis of pancreatic cancer. In a recent meta-analysis of 33 studies, Wang et al. [12] reported a pooled sensitivity of 91 % (95 % CI, 0.88–0.93) and a pooled specificity of 81 % (95 % CI, 0.75–0.85), slightly better than our results. Our results show that ^{18}F-FDG PET/CT imaging frequently led to a change in clinical staging, revealing extra-nodal involvement in 52.2 % of patients, and led to a change of management from surgery to adjuvant therapy due to unresectable pancreatic cancer. So it is important to stress that in 44 patients with ^{18}F-FDG PET/CT-positive lesions, the possibility of PET/CT-guided biopsy performed in 43 (given that one patient deceased shortly after) was extremely relevant for confirming malignancy of the pancreatic lesions. SUV did not help for differentiating malignant from nonmalignant lesions due to the known overlap in ^{18}F-FDG uptake. The PET/CT-guided biopsy is especially useful in patients where the clinical history is confusing [13, 14], for example, patients with chronic pancreatitis who develop changes in their symptomatology.

^{18}F-FDG PET/CT provides metabolic information and helps guide the biopsy to the region with the highest metabolism, increasing the likelihood to have a representative histological sample. In our experience, adequate histological material was obtained in 94.4 % (34/36) of patients. Two biopsy attempts were not successful on the first try; both cases were part of the 51.4 % patients in which ^{18}F-FDG PET/CT revealed extra-nodal involvement (both presented hepatic lesions with high ^{18}F-FDG uptake). The diagnosis was made by biopsy of these metastatic lesions, which are usually easier to access than primary pancreatic lesion. The accuracy of ^{18}F-FDG for staging pancreatic cancer is also well documented [1, 4, 10, 11, 15]. Although extra-nodal involvement implies unresectability of the tumor, the biopsy is still necessary to guide chemotherapy [1]

The complication rate associated with PET/CT-guided biopsy was 5.6 % of our patients (2/36), all cases being peripancreatic hematoma. There was no mortality related to the procedure. Other investigators also found low complication rates for pancreatic percutaneous guided biopsy [7, 8, 16–18]. However, patients are exposed to radiation.

The proper management of patients with pancreatic cancer requires a multidisciplinary approach, in which the access to modern imaging techniques is essential.

Case 7.1
^{18}F-FDG PET falsely negative in pancreatic adenocarcinoma

Clinical history: A 61-year-old male presented with recent onset of diarrhea, diabetes mellitus type II, weight loss, lipidic malabsorption, and a plasma level of Ca 19–9 of 60 IU/ml (Fig. 7.1).

Imaging procedures:

CECT: There is a lesion in the head of the pancreas (4 × 3 cm) infiltrating mesenteric and splenoportal vessels. The canal of Wirsung is dilated. There are bilateral lung metastases (the more prominent is displayed at the right lung basis).

EUS: There is a lesion in the head of the pancreas, hypoechoic, with irregular margins, and no fat plane between the lesion and the superior mesenteric and splenic vessels. The canal of Wirsung is dilated.

^{18}F-FDG PET/CT: The lesion in the head of the pancreas and pulmonary metastases showed no significant ^{18}F-FDG metabolism. However, the lung nodules are below PET resolution.

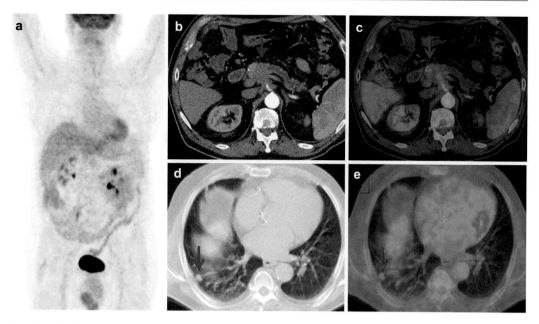

Fig. 7.1 ¹⁸F-FDG PET maximum intensity projection (**a**). Axial CECT (arterial phase) demonstrates a 3 cm hypodense lesion in the head of the pancreas with ill-defined margins and infiltrates the superior mesenteric artery (**b**, *red arrow*). The axial ¹⁸F-FDG PET/CECT (arterial phase) co-registration better demonstrates the absence of significant ¹⁸F-FDG uptake in the pancreatic lesion (**c**, *red arrow*). A low-dose CT documents multiple, bilateral lung metastases, the largest one in the right lung base (**d**, *red arrow*), showing no significant uptake on the fused image (**e**, *red arrow*), but they are at the limits of PET resolution

Histological examination (EUS-guided FNA): Mucinous adenocarcinoma with low cellularity.

Recommendations: ¹⁸F-FDG PET/CT is not helpful for mucinous adenocarcinoma with low cellularity.

Case 7.2

Uncommon pancreatic NHL (high-grade B-cell lymphoma with features intermediate between diffuse large B-cell lymphoma and Burkitt lymphoma)

Clinical history: A 41-year-old male presented with biliary and pancreatic obstructive syndrome and worsening abdominal pain. US and CT demonstrate a mass originating from the head of the pancreas. FNA: B-cell lymphoproliferative disorder (CD20+) (Fig. 7.2).

¹⁸F-FDG PET/CT: Co-registered ¹⁸F-FDG PET and CECT (arterial phase).

Heterogeneous hypodense bulky mass (10 × 6 cm), intensely ¹⁸F-FDG-avid (SUVmax = 18.5), arising from the head of the pancreas, encasing

the common bile duct (internal biliary stent visible). There is aerobilia and mild intrahepatic duct dilation. Photopenic areas likely represent necrosis.

Interpretation: ¹⁸F-FDG PET/CT consistent with high-grade pancreatic lymphoma (stage IE with abdominal bulky).

Histological examination (US-guided FNAB): High-grade B-cell lymphoma with features intermediate between diffuse large B-cell lymphoma and Burkitt lymphoma (FISH c-myc amplification via t(8;22) translocation). Bone marrow biopsy was negative for lymphomatous infiltration.

Recommendations: ¹⁸F-FDG PET/CT is helpful for staging high-grade NHL.

Case 7.3

Granulomatous pancreatitis

Clinical history: A 57-year-old male with a history of Hodgkin disease presented with back pain. The plasma levels of CEA and Ca19-9 were normal (Fig. 7.3).

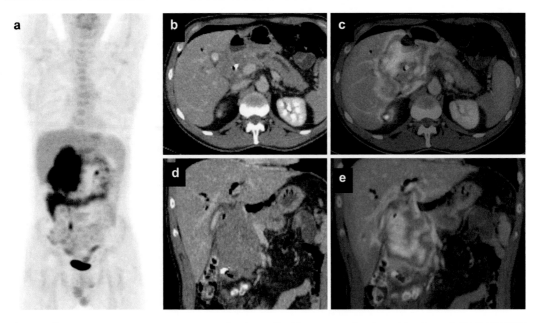

Fig. 7.2 ¹⁸F-FDG PET maximum intensity projection (**a**). Axial CECT – venous phase (**b**). Axial ¹⁸F-FDG PET/CECT – venous phase co-registration (**c**). Coronal CECT – pancreatic phase (**d**). Coronal ¹⁸F-FDG PET/CECT – venous phase co-registration (**e**)

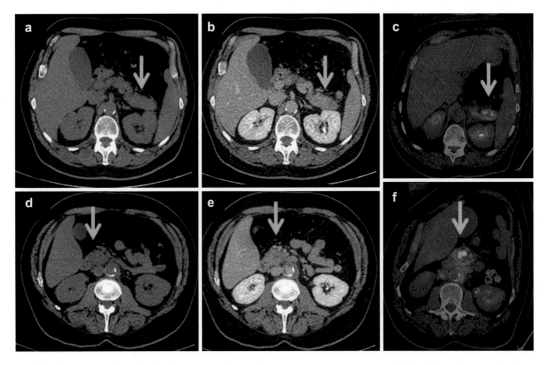

Fig. 7.3 Unenhanced CT demonstrates the pancreatic tail lesion (**a**), venous phase of the tail lesion (**b**), and ¹⁸F-FDG PET/CT demonstrates intense glycolytic activity in the head of the pancreas (**c**). Unenhanced CT dem-onstrates the pancreatic head lesion (**d**), venous phase of the head lesion (**e**), and ¹⁸F-FDG PET/CT demonstrates intense glycolytic activity in the pancreatic tail lesion (**f**)

Imaging procedures:

CECT: Hypovascular lesion in the head of the pancreas ($4 \times 2.5 \times 4.3$ cm) in all contrast phases. A similar lesion (5.5×2.4 cm) is seen in the tail of the pancreas. There is no evidence of vascular infiltration and no dilation of pancreatic ducts.

^{18}F-FDG PET/CT demonstrates two areas of intense and heterogeneous ^{18}F-FDG uptake in the head (SUVmax = 23.0) and tail of the pancreas (SUVmax = 17.0) consistent with a multifocal pancreatic neoplasm.

Histological examination (after spleno-pancreatectomy)*:* Extensive inflammatory necrotizing granulomatous process and diffuse granulomatous necrotizing vasculitis (small and medium vessels).

Recommendations: ^{18}F-FDG PET/CT is helpful to differentiate between benign and malignant pancreatic processes . However, granulomatous lesions are false positive.

Case 7.4
Malignant transformation of intraductal papillary mucinous neoplasm (IPMN) with hepatic metastases

Clinical history: A 60-year-old male presented with a 3-month history of refractory gastric pain, lack of appetite, and 4 kg weight loss. US and CT demonstrated three pancreatic cystic lesions. The plasma level of CA19-9 was increased (Fig. 7.4).

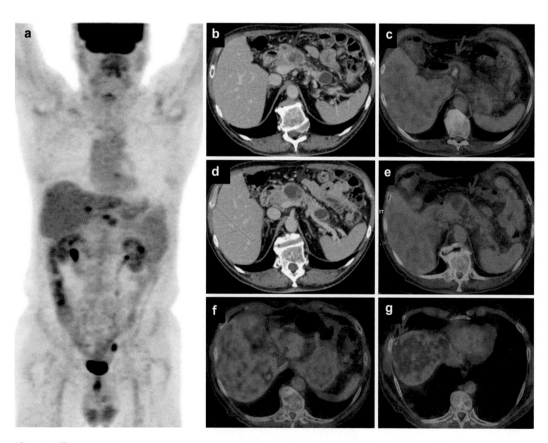

Fig. 7.4 ^{18}F-FDG PET maximum intensity projection (MIP) (**a**). CECT (pancreatic phase): solid component of the cystic lesion in the body of the pancreas (**b**). ^{18}F-FDG PET/CT demonstrates increased uptake in the solid component of the lesion (**c**). CECT (pancreatic phase): lateral extension of the solid component of the lesion in the body of the pancreas (**d**). ^{18}F-FDG PET/CT demonstrates intense uptake at the same level (**e**); and ^{18}F-FDG PET/CT: two ^{18}F-FDG-avid liver metastases (**f, g**)

Imaging procedures:

CECT: There is a cystic lesion (4.5 × 3.2 cm) with a solid component in the body of the pancreas with obstruction and dilatation of the Wirsung duct. The lesion is adjacent to the celiac axis and adheres to the spleno-mesenteric confluence and duodenal bulb. Two more cystic lesions are present in the body (2.3 × 1.8 cm) and tail (3.5 × 2.5 cm) of the pancreas. This radiological pattern is consistent with type II IPMN with malignant degeneration of the body lesion.

There is a 1 cm ill-defined lesion in segment VII of the liver close to the inferior vena cava, hypodense in all contrast phases of the CT that needs further assessment with ^{18}F-FDG PET/CT.

^{18}F-FDG PET/CT: ^{18}F-FDG uptake is seen in the solid part of the cystic lesion in the body of the pancreas (SUVmax = 4.5). Two small lesions are seen in the segment VII and dome of the liver (SUVmax = 3.5), respectively.

Interpretation: ^{18}F-FDG-avid neoplastic process likely pancreatic primary with hepatic metastases.

Histological examination (US-FNA of the hepatic lesion): Moderately differentiated adenocarcinoma.

Recommendations: ^{18}F-FDG PET/CT can help differentiate benign and malignant pancreatic lesions. In this case, PET clearly detected the area of IPMN degeneration. In addition, ^{18}F-FDG PET/CT demonstrated ^{18}F-FDG uptake in two hepatic lesions and detected an additional small lesion in the dome of the liver.

Case 7.5

Moderately differentiated pancreatic neuroendocrine tumor (NET) with hepatic metastases

Clinical history: A 67-year-old male presented with a recent diagnosis of moderately differentiated neuroendocrine tumor (NET) of the pancreatic tail and with hepatic metastases documented by conventional imaging (Figs. 7.5 and 7.6).

Imaging Procedures

^{18}F-FDG PET/CT: Intense ^{18}F-FDG uptake in the region of the tail of the pancreas consistent with known primary NET. Multiple ^{18}F-FDG-avid, hypodense hepatic metastases, some displaying central photopenic areas, likely due to central necrosis.

^{68}Ga]DOTANOC PET/CT: Demonstrates mild uptake in a solitary peripancreatic node on the

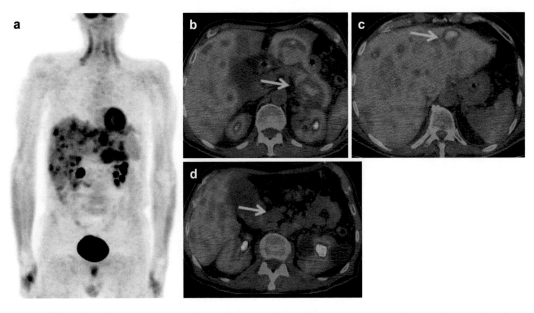

Fig. 7.5 ^{18}F-FDG PET maximum intensity projection (MIP) (**a**); axial ^{18}F-FDG PET/CT shows an area of moderately increased tracer uptake in the tail of the pancreas (**b**, *green arrow*) and multiple ^{18}F-FDG-avid hepatic lesions (**c**, *green arrow*). A solitary peripancreatic node on the midline does not show any abnormal ^{18}F-FDG uptake (**d**, *green arrow*)

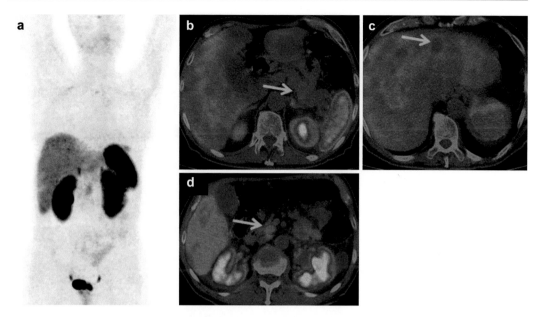

Fig. 7.6 [⁶⁸Ga]DOTANOC maximum intensity projection (MIP) (**a**); axial [⁶⁸Ga]DOTANOC PET/CT at the same level as ¹⁸F-FDG PET shows no significant tracer uptake at the primary site (**b**, *green arrow*) nor at hepatic lesions (**c**, *green arrow*); however, the same solitary peripancreatic node on the midline demonstrates mild SSTR expression (**d**, *green arrow*)

midline and no significant somatostatin receptors (SSTR) expression at any other site.

Histological examination (US-FNAB of the hepatic lesion in the segment III): Moderately differentiated neuroendocrine tumor (G2-NET sec. WHO 2010, Ki-67 = 19.6 %) with central necrosis.

Recommendations: The combination of [⁶⁸Ga]DOTANOC and ¹⁸F-FDG PET/CT for staging NET patients allows evaluation of tumor heterogeneity (i.e., aggressiveness and somatostatin receptor expression status). These procedures are complementary for staging, have a prognostic value, and provide guidance for the choice of therapy.

Case 7.6
Pancreatic carcinoma

Clinical history: A 60-year-old male presented with a recent diagnosis of a large pancreatic lesion by conventional imaging (Fig. 7.7).

¹⁸F-FDG PET/CT: Intense uptake is seen in the head of the pancreas (SUVmax = 6.5). No other lesions are seen.

Interpretation: ¹⁸F-FDG-avid neoplastic process likely primary pancreatic cancer.

Histological examination (PET/CT-guided biopsy of the pancreatic lesion): Moderately differentiated adenocarcinoma.

Recommendations: ¹⁸F-FDG PET/CT can help differentiate benign and malignant pancreatic lesions and can guide biopsy to the most metabolically active part of the lesion.

Case 7.7
Acute pancreatitis

Clinical history: A 64-year-old female presented with a large pancreatic lesion seen on conventional imaging (Fig. 7.8).

¹⁸F-FDG PET/CT: Intense ¹⁸F-FDG uptake is seen in the head of the pancreas (SUVmax = 9.5).

Interpretation: ¹⁸F-FDG-avid neoplastic process likely pancreatic primary.

Histological examination (PET/CT-guided biopsy of the pancreatic lesion): Acute pancreatitis.

Recommendations: Inflammatory processes are ¹⁸F-FDG-avid, and ¹⁸F-FDG PET/CT can guide biopsy for histological examination and differentiation of benign inflammatory processes and malignant lesions.

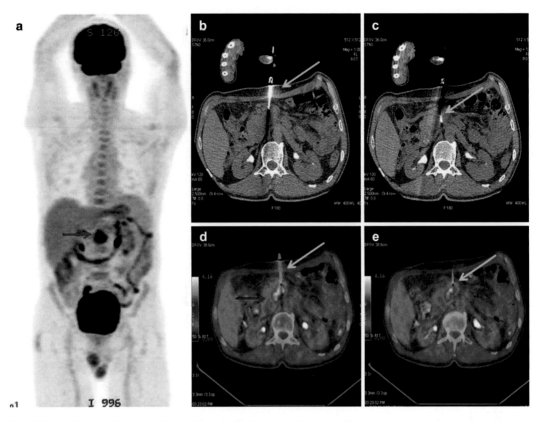

Fig. 7.7 A 60-year-old male patient with a pancreatic lesion was referred for ¹⁸F-FDG PET/CT. Maximum intensity projection (MIP) image (**a**) shows intense uptake in the head of the pancreas (*red arrow*). The placement of the biopsy needle in the lesion is demonstrated on the axial CT images (**b**, **c**). The axial fusion image of PET/CT images (**d**, **e**) confirms the location of the needle (*blue arrow*) in the metabolic lesion (*red arrow*)

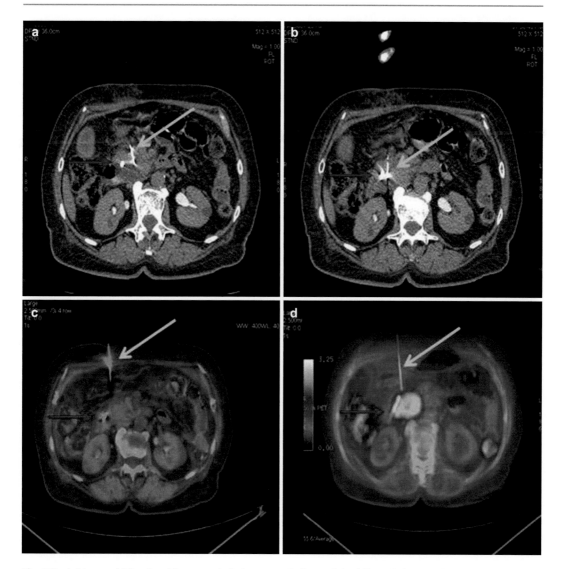

Fig. 7.8 A 64-year-old female with pancreatic lesion was referred to ¹⁸F-FDG PET/CT. The axial CT images (**a**, **b**) demonstrate the placement of the needle (*blue arrow*) in the lesion and the biliary drainage catheter (*red arrow*). The axial fusion image of PET/CT images (**c**, **d**) confirms the location of the needle (*blue arrow*) in the metabolic lesion

References

1. Anderson KE, Mack T, Silverman D. Cancer of the pancreas. In: Schottenfeld D, Fraumeni Jr JF, editors. Cancer epidemiology and prevention. 3rd ed. New York: Oxford University Press; 2006.
2. Zech C, Helmberger T, Wichmann M, Holzknecht N, Diebold J, Reiser MF. Large core biopsy of the pancreas under CT fluoroscopy control: results and complications. J Comput Assist Tomogr. 2002;26(5):743–9.
3. Itani K, Taylor T, Green L. Needle biopsy for suspicious lesions of the head of the pancreas: pitfalls and implications for therapy. J Gastrointest Surg. 1997;1(4):337–41.
4. National Comprehensive Cancer Network. NCCN clinical practice guidelines in oncology. Pancreatic Adenocarcinoma. 2013;1. Available at http://www.nccn.org/professionals/physician_gls/pdf/pancreatic.pdf.
5. Raczynski S, Teich N, Borte G, Wittenburg H, Mossner J, Caca K. Percutaneous transgastric irrigation drainage in combination with endoscopic necrosectomy in necrotizing pancreatitis (with videos). Gastrointest Endosc. 2006;64(3):420–4.
6. Mueller PR, Miketic L, Simeone J, Silverman S, Saini S, Wittenberg J, et al. Severe acute pancreatitis after

percutaneous biopsy of the pancreas. AJR Am J Roentgenol. 1988;151(3):493–4.

7. Tseng HS, Chen CY, Chan WP, et al. Percutaneous transgastric computed tomography-guided biopsy of the pancreas using large needles. World J Gastroenterol. 2009;15:5972–5.

8. Paulsen SD, Nghiem HV, Negussie E, Higgins EJ, Caoili EM, Francis IR. Evaluation of imaging-guided core biopsy of pancreatic masses. AJR Am J Roentgenol. 2006;187(3):769–72.

9. Farma JM, Santillan AA, Melis M, Walters J, Belinc D, Chen DT, et al. PET/CT fusion scan enhances CT staging in patients with pancreatic neoplasms. Ann Surg Oncol. 2008;15(9):2465–71.

10. Kauhanen S, et al. Positron emission tomography in the diagnosis and staging of pancreatic and neuroendocrine tumors. 2009.

11. Sahani DV, Bonaffini PA, Catalano OA, Guimaraes AR, Blake MA. State-of-the-art PET/CT of the pancreas: current role and emerging indications. Radiographics. 2012;32(4):1133–58; discussion 1158–60.

12. Wang Z, Chen JQ, Liu JL, Qin XG, Huang Y. FDG-PET in diagnosis, staging and prognosis of pancreatic carcinoma: a meta-analysis. World J Gastroenterol. 2013;19(29):4808–17. doi:10.3748/wjg.v19.i29.4808.

13. Kauhanen SP, Komar G, Seppänen MP, Dean KI, Minn HR, Kajander SA, Rinta-Kiikka I, Alanen K, Borra RJ, Puolakkainen PA, Nuutila P, Ovaska JT. A prospective diagnostic accuracy study of 18F-fluorodeoxyglucose positron emission tomography/computed tomography, multidetector row computed tomography, and magnetic resonance imaging in primary diagnosis and staging of pancreatic cancer. Ann Surg. 2009;250(6):957–63.

14. Keogan MT, Tyler D, Clark L, Branch MS, McDermott VG, DeLong DM, Coleman RE. Diagnosis of pancreatic carcinoma: role of FDG PET. AJR Am J Roentgenol. 1998;171(6):1565–70.

15. Delbeke D, Rose DM, Chapman WC, Pinson CW, Wright JK, Beauchamp RD, Shyr Y, Leach SD. Optimal interpretation of FDG PET in the diagnosis, staging and management of pancreatic carcinoma. J Nucl Med. 1999;40(11):1784–91.

16. Li L, Liu LZ, Wu QL, Mo YX, Liu XW, Cui CY, Wan DS. CT-guided core needle biopsy in the diagnosis of pancreatic diseases with an automated biopsy gun. J Vasc Interv Radiol. 2008;19(1):89–94.

17. Chiang Jeng TYNG, et al. Computed tomography-guided percutaneous biopsy of pancreatic masses using pneumodissection. Radiol Bras [online]. 2013;46(3):139–42 [cited 2013-09-25].

18. Erturk SM, Mortelé KJ, Tuncali K, Saltzman JR, Lao R, Silverman SG. Fine-needle aspiration biopsy of solid pancreatic masses: comparison of CT and endoscopic sonography guidance. AJR Am J Roentgenol. 2006;187(6):1531–5.

18F-FDG PET/CT for Bone and Soft Tissue Biopsy

8

Cristina Nanni, Elena Tabacchi, and Stefano Fanti

8.1 Overview

In the clinical practice, it is quite common to diagnose a lesion in the bone or soft tissues that is amenable to biopsy. This is particularly true in patients who come to the hospital with a history of cancer, with radiological signs consistent with malignancy, or with the suspicion of focal septic inflammation.

Frequently, these conditions cannot be clearly distinguished on the basis of noninvasive imaging procedures such as US, ceCT, MR, or even PET/CT. This is particularly relevant from a clinical point of view since the therapeutic approach as well as the prognosis is different for a malignant lesion, for a benign lesion, or for an inflammatory or infectious process.

Open incisional biopsy (OIB) was traditionally the method of choice for diagnosing tumors and tumorlike lesions of the musculoskeletal system. It usually requires hospitalization of 48 ± 72 h, an operating room (time and personnel), and general anesthesia. While OIB is still considered the gold standard because of its accuracy (close to 100 %), it is associated with several drawbacks, including morbidity and surgical complications, the risk of tumor contamination of surrounding normal soft tissues (an important issue for future limb-sparing surgery), and high cost. The development of imaging-guided biopsies for musculoskeletal lesions (computed tomography, ultrasound, and fluoroscopy) has mostly overcome these disadvantages. It is especially suitable for sites that are deep or difficult to reach such as the spine and to avoid injury to major vessels or nerves [1].

In recent years, it became evident that CT-guided core-needle biopsy is safe, easy to perform, efficient, and less invasive than open incisional biopsy. It should therefore be considered as a first-line biopsy procedure for musculoskeletal lesions.

The performance of CT-guided core-needle biopsy is more than acceptable, as is the accuracy in distinguishing benign from malignant lesions, the accuracy in distinguishing low- from high-grade sarcomas, the accuracy for specific diagnosis, the repeated biopsy rate, and the complication rate. The performance for specific diagnosis is generally higher for bone than soft tissue lesions for both CT-guided core-needle biopsy and incisional biopsy [2–7].

No significant risks in terms of local recurrence along the core-needle biopsy tract have been reported [8].

However, the performance of CT-guided core-needle biopsy for specific diagnosis of benign soft tissue tumors as well as infection and

C. Nanni (✉) • E. Tabacchi • S. Fanti
Nuclear Medicine, AOU Policlinico S.Orsola-
Malpighi, Bologna, Italy
e-mail: cristina.nanni@aosp.bo.it; tabacchielena@
libero.it; stefano.fanti@aosp.bo.it

© Springer International Publishing 2016
J. Cerci et al. (eds.), *Oncological PET/CT with Histological Confirmation*,
DOI 10.1007/978-3-319-27880-3_8

inflammation is relatively low [2]: even with a correct procedure, the biopsy is diagnostic in only 48–78 % of patients.

Furthermore, once the biopsy has been done and adequate material is obtained, the antibiogram of an infected tissue is reliable in only approximately half of the patients [9–11], and this is crucial to choose the most efficient antibiotic therapy.

The CT-guided biopsy may not be diagnostic due to sampling error. The role of functional imaging such as ¹⁸F-FDG PET/CT is to drive the biopsy toward the most metabolically active area of a lesion. ¹⁸F-FDG PET/CT imaging can be employed offline or as a direct guide. As an offline method, ¹⁸F-FDG PET/CT transaxial images can be compared side by side to the diagnostic CT images acquired during the CT-guided biopsy, and the needle can be visually guided into the most metabolically active area. This process can be done everywhere, even in hospital where PET/CT tomographs are not available. However, since this procedure is only visual, mistakes can be done especially in case of large and partially necrotic masses.

The direct use of a PET/CT tomograph to guide the biopsy is much more reliable in terms of biopsy accuracy. PET/CT images allow identification of the most active lesion (if more than one are detected) and to sample the most active tissue within the target lesion.

The acquisition of a PET/CT image during the procedure to verify the correct position of the needle is feasible with last-generation scanners, which can acquire images in a very short time lapse (1 min/bed position on a 3D tomograph).

Soft tissue and bone lesions requiring histological examination are basically oncological and infectious processes. Among oncological processes, soft tissue sarcomas and bone sarcomas are the most common that are ¹⁸F-FDG-avid. The most common types are fibrosarcoma and malignant fibrous histiocytoma among those originating from fibrous tissue; liposarcoma originating from fatty tissue; leiomyosarcoma from smooth muscle; rhabdomyosarcoma from skeletal muscle; angiosarcoma, lymphangiosarcoma, and Kaposi sarcoma from blood and lymph vessels;

hemangiopericytoma from perivascular tissue; synovial sarcoma from synovial tissue; schwannoma from peripheral nerves; and gastrointestinal stromal tumor (GIST) from mesenchymal cells. Bone sarcomas are less common and include Ewing sarcoma and osteosarcoma. There are multiple indications to perform a PET scan in patients affected by sarcomas. Several articles have demonstrated the role of ¹⁸F-FDG PET and PET/CT not only as a guide for biopsy but also for predicting the prognosis, for staging and restaging the disease, and for assessing the response to therapy [12, 13–25]. PET is also useful to differentiate benign fluid collections from soft tissue sarcomas [26]. Multiple myeloma and suspected bone metastases from other primary tumors are also indication biopsy.

Among inflammatory/infectious diseases, suspicion of spondylodiscitis, tuberculous bone infection, and prosthetic bone infection are the most common indications for bone biopsy. Differentiation of infection from aseptic inflammation and the identification of the pathogen have major therapeutic implications [9].

Case 8.1
Clinical history

A 17-year-old man with a history of tuberculosis underwent whole body ¹⁸F-FDG PET/CT showing multiple foci of uptake in the bones, inconsistent with the clinical status of the patient.

¹⁸F-FDG PET/CT-guided biopsy was performed on one of the most metabolically active lesion, in the right iliac bone, to exclude a concomitant bone lymphoma.

Histopathology demonstrated tuberculosis.

Only one biopsy was sufficient to reach a diagnosis.

No complications were reported.

Findings

Several focal uptake in lymph nodes, soft tissues, and bones.

Teaching point

The patient was positioned in the prone position, and biopsy was performed by direct access (B, C) with an 18G needle in a lesion with higher ¹⁸F-FDG uptake (C) and safe location. Indeed, in patients with multiple lesions, PET/CT allows

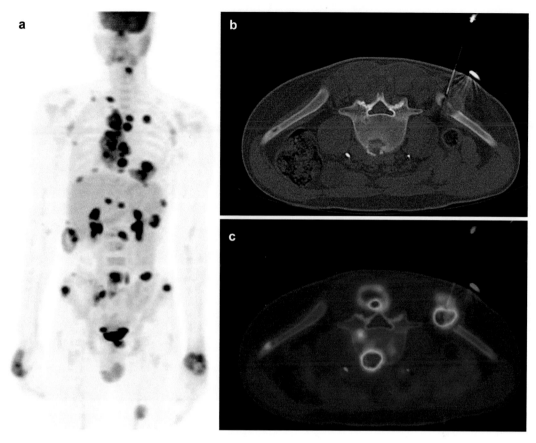

Fig. 8.1 (**a**) MIP; (**b**) CT scan; (**c**) PET/CT scan, transaxial view

not only the identification of the lesions with the higher metabolism but also the identification of the most accessible site for biopsy with reduction of sampling errors and risks of complications.

Recommendations

Because the glucose metabolism is also elevated in activated inflammatory cells, nonmalignant inflammatory conditions are also 18F-FDG-avid.

In some cases, it is not possible to differentiate infectious processes from malignancy because of their similar morphology. For example, granulomatous infection with central necrosis or cavitation may appear indistinguishable from a centrally necrotic or cavitating neoplasm, and biopsy is necessary for diagnosis (Fig. 8.1).

Case 8.2

Clinical history

A 37-year-old female with a history of right thigh sarcoma was treated with chemotherapy in 2011.

She presented with persistent pain in her right thigh associating with a discharging fistula, and 18F-FDG PET/CT was performed.

PET-guided biopsy was directed to the most 18F-FDG-avid site, leading to histological confirmation of sarcoma recurrence.

Findings: focal uptake in the medial region of the right thigh.

Teaching point

Patient was positioned in the supine position with legs immobilized, and biopsy was performed with direct access of soft tissue lesion with an 18G needle (B and C). Single-bed position of 18F-FDG PET/CT (D and E) was acquired to confirm needle position in an area with 18F-FDG uptake. Special attention should be kept to avoid the puncture of major femoral vessels,

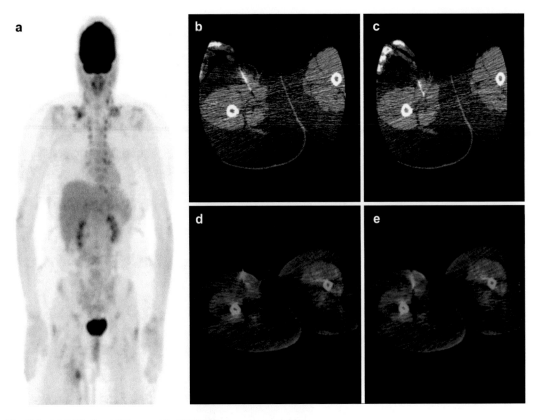

Fig. 8.2 (**a**) MIP; (**b**, **c**) TC scan; (**d**, **e**) PET/CT scan, transaxial image

but in this case, this risk was low due to the peripheral location of the lesion.

Recommendation: Focal ¹⁸F-FDG PET/CT uptake in soft tissue can be related not only to neoplastic lesions like sarcoma but also to inflammatory/infective disease. For this reason, before biopsy, it is important to consider the patient's history (Fig. 8.2).

Case 8.3

Clinical history

This 68-year-old male presented with a left thigh swelling and severe pain.

On conventional imaging, a soft tissue mass was identified and encased and eroded the left acetabulum.

Histological analysis of the PET-guided biopsy to the most hypermetabolic site showed DLBCL.

Findings: intense ¹⁸F-FDG uptake in the proximal region of the thigh, extended from the left iliac fossa to the proximal third of thigh.

Teaching point

The patient was positioned in the supine position with pelvis immobilized. Direct access to the lesion with highest ¹⁸F-FDG uptake (D and E) and safest path (lower risk of local complication like puncture of abdominal organs or major vessels) was chosen for biopsy (B and C) using an 18G needle.

The needle was placed along the planned surgical access for resecting the lesion due to the possibility of tumor cell seeding along the needle tract. Even if the relationship between biopsy and later recurrence is difficult to confirm, it is sometimes considered a major contraindication. This potential complication of biopsy procedures needs to be discussed with the patient during the informed consent process.

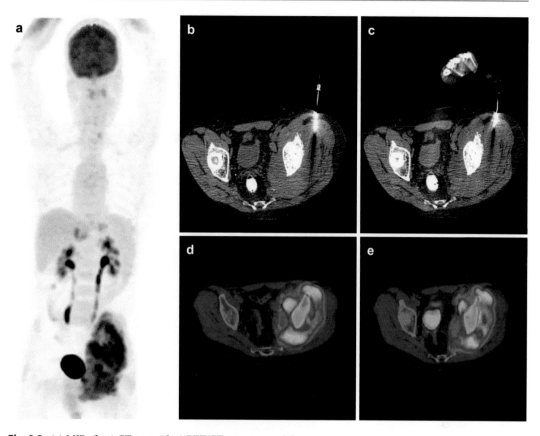

Fig. 8.3 (**a**) MIP; (**b**, **c**) CT scan; (**d**, **e**) PET/CT scan, transaxial

Recommendations: ¹⁸F-FDG PET/CT can be useful to identify the optimal site for biopsy (in terms of highest uptake and safety access) for histological confirmation of the disease process. ¹⁸F-FDG PET/CT is also useful for staging, restaging, and evaluation of response to treatment (Fig. 8.3).

Case 8.4

Clinical history

This 61-year-old female was complaining of severe pain to her left foot.

A PET-guided biopsy of the shown hypermetabolic medial forefoot lesion led to the diagnosis of chondrosarcoma.

Findings: focal uptake in the left medial forefoot lesion at the level of the first metatarsophalangeal articulation.

Findings

The patient was positioned in the prone position with immobilization of the feet. Biopsy was performed by direct access (B and C) of the most hypermetabolic site of lesion (D and E) with an 18G needle.

In this case, due to the distal location of the lesion, there is no risk to injure organs or major vessels, even if there is formation of postprocedure hematoma. It is important to perform a manual compression soon after the needle removal.

Recommendations

The path of a future surgery should be considered to access the biopsy (Fig. 8.4).

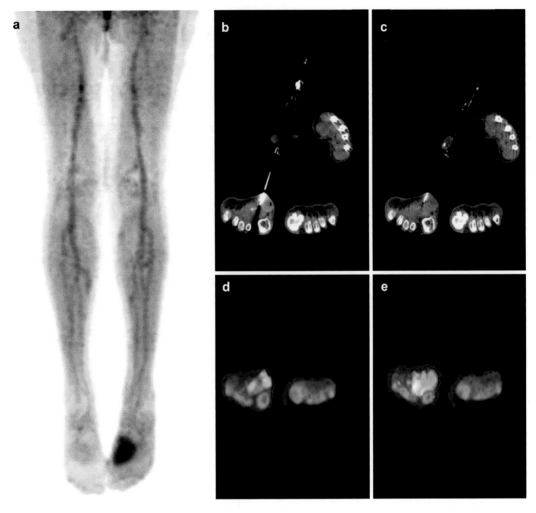

Fig. 8.4 (**a**) MIP; (**b**, **c**) CT scan; (**d**, **e**) PET/CT scan, transaxial

References

1. Issakov J, Flusser G, Kollender Y, Merimsky O, Lifschitz-Mercer B, Meller I. Computed tomography-guided core needle biopsy for bone and soft tissue tumors. Isr Med Assoc J. 2003;5(1):28–30.
2. Kiatisevi P, Thanakit V, Sukunthanak B, Boonthatip M, Bumrungchart S, Witoonchart K. Computed tomography-guided core needle biopsy versus incisional biopsy in diagnosing musculoskeletal lesions. J Orthop Surg (Hong Kong). 2013;21(2):204–8.
3. Koscick RL, Petersilge CA, Makley JT, Abdul-Karim FW. CT-guided fine needle aspiration and needle core biopsy of skeletal lesions. Complementary diagnostic techniques. Acta Cytol. 1998;42(3):697–702.
4. Jelinek JS, Murphey MD, Welker JA, Henshaw RM, Kransdorf MJ, Shmookler BM, et al. Diagnosis of primary bone tumors with image-guided percutaneous biopsy: experience with 110 tumors. Radiology. 2002;223(3):731–7.
5. Holzapfel BM, Ludemann M, Holzapfel DE, Rechl H, Rudert M. Open biopsy of bone and soft tissue tumors: guidelines for precise surgical procedures. Oper Orthop Traumatol. 2012;24(4–5):403–15; quiz 416–7.
6. Ferguson KB, McGlynn J, Jane M, Ritchie D, Mahendra A. Outcome of image-guided biopsies: retrospective review of the west of Scotland musculoskeletal oncology service. Surgeon. 2014. pii: S1479–666X(14)00119-X. doi: 10.1016/j.surge.2014.09.002. [Epub ahead of print].
7. Toomayan GA, Major NM. Utility of CT-guided biopsy of suspicious skeletal lesions in patients with known primary malignancies. AJR Am J Roentgenol. 2011;196(2):416–23.
8. Saghieh S, Masrouha KZ, Musallam KM, Mahfouz R, Abboud M, Khoury NJ, et al. The risk of local recur-

rence along the core-needle biopsy tract in patients with bone sarcomas. Iowa Orthop J. 2010;30:80–3.

9. Gasbarrini A, Boriani L, Salvadori C, Mobarec S, Kreshak J, Nanni C, et al. Biopsy for suspected spondylodiscitis. Eur Rev Med Pharmacol Sci. 2012;16 Suppl 2:26–34.

10. Gasbarrini A, Boriani L, Nanni C, Zamparini E, Rorato G, Ghermandi R, et al. Spinal infection multidisciplinary management project (SIMP): from diagnosis to treatment guideline. Int J Immunopathol Pharmacol. 2011;24(1 Suppl 2):95–100.

11. Gouliouris T, Aliyu SH, Brown NM. Spondylodiscitis: update on diagnosis and management. J Antimicrob Chemother. 2010;65 Suppl 3:iii11–24.

12. Toner GC, Hicks RJ. PET for sarcomas other than gastrointestinal stromal tumors. Oncologist. 2008;13 Suppl 2:22–6.

13. Benz MR, Czernin J, Allen-Auerbach MS, Tap WD, Dry SM, Elashoff D, et al. FDG-PET/CT imaging predicts histopathologic treatment responses after the initial cycle of neoadjuvant chemotherapy in high-grade soft-tissue sarcomas. Clin Cancer Res. 2009; 15(8):2856–63.

14. Benz MR, Czernin J, Tap WD, Eckardt JJ, Seeger LL, Allen-Auerbach MS, et al. FDG-PET/CT imaging predicts histopathologic treatment responses after neoadjuvant therapy in adult primary bone sarcomas. Sarcoma. 2010;2010:143540.

15. Benz MR, Tchekmedyian N, Eilber FC, Federman N, Czernin J, Tap WD. Utilization of positron emission tomography in the management of patients with sarcoma. Curr Opin Oncol. 2009;21(4):345–51.

16. Borbely K, Nemeth Z, Kasler M. Clinical application of 18F-FDG PET/CT in the treatment of sarcomas. Magy Onkol. 2014;58(1):24–31.

17. Ceyssens S, Stroobants S. Sarcoma. Methods Mol Biol (Clifton NJ). 2011;727:191–203.

18. Charest M, Hickeson M, Lisbona R, Novales-Diaz J-A, Derbekyan V, Turcotte RE. FDG PET/CT imaging in primary osseous and soft tissue sarcomas: a retrospective review of 212 cases. Eur J Nucl Med Mol Imaging. 2009;36(12):1944–51.

19. Costelloe CM, Raymond AK, Fitzgerald NE, Mawlawi OR, Nunez RF, Madewell JE, et al. Tumor necrosis in osteosarcoma: inclusion of the point of greatest metabolic activity from F-18 FDG PET/CT in the histopathologic analysis. Skeletal Radiol. 2010;39(2):131–40.

20. Dimitrakopoulou-Strauss A, Strauss LG, Egerer G, Vasamiliette J, Schmitt T, Haberkorn U, et al. Prediction of chemotherapy outcome in patients with metastatic soft tissue sarcomas based on dynamic FDG PET (dPET) and a multiparameter analysis. Eur J Nucl Med Mol Imaging. 2010;37(8):1481–9.

21. Eary JF, Hawkins DS, Rodler ET, Conrad 3rd EU. (18)F-FDG PET in sarcoma treatment response imaging. Am J Nucl Med Mol Imaging. 2011;1(1): 47–53.

22. Ferrari S, Balladelli A, Palmerini E, Vanel D. Imaging in bone sarcomas. The chemotherapist's point of view. Eur J Radiol. 2013;82(12):2076–82.

23. Herrmann K, Benz MR, Czernin J, Allen-Auerbach MS, Tap WD, Dry SM, et al. 18F-FDG-PET/CT Imaging as an early survival predictor in patients with primary high-grade soft tissue sarcomas undergoing neoadjuvant therapy. Clin Cancer Res. 2012; 18(7):2024–31.

24. Im HJ, Kim TS, Park S-Y, Min HS, Kim JH, Kang HG, et al. Prediction of tumour necrosis fractions using metabolic and volumetric 18F-FDG PET/CT indices, after one course and at the completion of neoadjuvant chemotherapy, in children and young adults with osteosarcoma. Eur J Nucl Med Mol Imaging. 2012;39(1):39–49.

25. Kolesnikov-Gauthier H, Leblond P, Rocourt N, Carpentier P. Contribution of FDG-PET in the management of pediatric sarcomas in 2011. Bull Cancer (Paris). 2011;98(5):501–14.

26. Amini B, Madewell JE, Chuang HH, Haygood TM, Hobbs BP, Fox PS, et al. Differentiation of benign fluid collections from soft-tissue sarcomas on. J Cancer. 2014;5(5):328–35.

Index